A plain speaking g

HEALTHY SKIN HEALTHY VIBES

Zaffrin O'Sullivan

Co-founder of Five Dot Botanics

Healthy Skin, Healthy Vibes © 2021

Copyright © Zaffrin O'Sullivan 2021

Cover Design by Natalie Chung

The content in this book is for information only and any opinion are the authors' own.

All Rights Reserved. No part of this publication maybe reproduced or transmitted in any form without prior permission.

ISBN: 978-1-5272-8283-4

For Hana, Noah + Eamonn

Contents

Introduction	vii
1 Skin Basics	1
2 Skin Care	42
3 The Beauty Industry	68
4 Decode Your Skincare	93
5 Skin & Wellness	112
6 Botanical Ingredients	132
Index	144

Introduction

I have always been interested in skin care. However, growing up the beauty industry wasn't one that resonated with me.

The skincare sections of department stores were bright places filled with immaculate women and often I didn't feel at ease visiting a beauty counter.

Glossy magazines were not particularly diverse, and they didn't represent the exciting breadth of people, races and faces I could see living in London.

The aspiration in skincare was to hold onto youthfulness. There wasn't much space for a more age inclusive conversation.

However, being interested in skin and particularly what it means to have healthy skin, never really went away. Even today, how I feel about myself links to how my skin is feelings and looking.

Over the years I have had blemishes, pigmentation, hormonal acne, pregnancy related skin issues, dehydrated skin, stressed skin and experimented with countless harsh products.

It turns out that I am not alone.

There are a lot of people like me who are interested in having healthy skin, that feel a bit out of place in the beauty aisles.

Despite feeling out of place within the beauty industry, I always wanted to create skincare products with a focus on skin health.

I am a lawyer by background and for many years behind the scenes I studied and researched how to develop, manufacture, and launch a personal cosmetic range.

Along the way I connected with a range of industry experts, gathering wisdom, insight and tips. I founded a global beauty community, Female Founders in Beauty, to help other women launch their own beauty brands and I am a passionate advocate for independent beauty brands.

After many years of research and partnering with an established and experienced cosmetic scientist, I launched Five Dot Botanics in 2019. We are a British minimal ingredient skincare company that makes skincare for all genders, ages, and races. We focus on plant-based ingredients and since launching we have picked up several beauty awards. It is great to see smaller indie brands gain recognition in the crowded beauty space.

Minimal ingredient skincare is not for everyone, some beauty fans are not interested in a "less is more" approach. However, I have always wanted to offer people the power of choice.

In my journey to launching a skincare company, I learned about all aspects of the beauty industry. I met cosmetic scientists, looked at formulations, visited labs, interrogated ingredients, read regulations, poured over cosmetic compliance documents, and discussed cosmetic safety as well as a lot more.

It has been a journey that has taught me a lot about skincare products, how they are made and what goes in them. Increasingly people are more interested in the ingredients contained in their personal cosmetics and offering consumers transparency and trust are key when it comes to skincare products.

I created this book as a simple plain-speaking guide for anyone who wants to learn about skin care, skin care routines and how skincare products are made and marketed.

As more people become interested in skin care, this book aims to offer an introduction to skin and supply easy to understand answers to a range of frequent questions related to skin, skincare and the beauty industry.

The aim of this book is to educate and empower a beginner to skincare and is written in an easy to understand format.

As an advocate for a more natural plant-based approach to skincare, this book approaches skin care with that lens in mind. This is not the only way to go when it comes to skin, however, it is an area that more people are becoming interested in.

I hope you enjoy this book and find it useful in helping you on our journey to healthy happy skin.

Zaffrin x

1 Skin Basics

Understanding your skin and its structure is an effective way to learn about the skin's functions and what skincare products do.

Skin care goes beyond how our skin looks, it is part of looking after ourselves. In our quest to have glowing skin or address specific cosmetic skin concerns, we can forget the role skin plays in our overall health. Our skin is an amazing organ and it deserves to be looked after. It is so important to have a good daily skin care routine, for best skin health. There are no fast fixes when it comes to supporting healthy skin, it is something that we should pay attention to consistently.

> *Having healthy skin is a lifelong process.*

Making good choices for the health of your skin are key for the long term. Preventing potential skin problems early is easier than trying to fix skin issues in the future.

Understanding skin can help us understand how our products, lifestyle and skin care routines affect the skin.

Why is skin important?

Skin is an organ and its primary function is protection.

When we think of major bodily organs, skin is rarely on the list. It is our most visible organ and the condition of our skin can tell a lot about us.

The colour, the evenness of tone, the smoothness, whether it's shiny or dull can all supply clues about our overall health and wellbeing.

Our skin condition can also be a source of anxiety and stress.

When we feel our skin doesn't look or feel how we want, it can affect our self-esteem and confidence.

Acne, blemishes, redness, irritation, age spots, wrinkles are just some of skin conditions people can feel uncomfortable about.

How we feel about our skin can go to the core of how we feel about ourselves.

The rise of photo filters and image editing apps has not helped, it has increased the idea of impossibly flawless skin, fuelling a rise in dissatisfaction with how our skin looks. We see ourselves or others with these filters and we can easily forget that the portrayal of skin through this lens is completely unreal.

Skin is important not just because of how it makes us look and feel. Skin is important because it is a vital protector of our overall health.

What does our skin do?

Our skin is not the same everywhere on our body and it takes on different thickness, colour, and texture all over our body. Our skin is constantly renewing itself and day to day our skin has several distinct functions including:

- Prevents water loss
- Prevents entry of bacteria
- Regulates temperature
- Stores water + fat
- Sensorial functions
- Helps to make vitamin D
- Helps protect us from the sun

Our skin serves as a protective shield against heat, light, injury, and infection and it plays a primary role in supporting our health. Thinking about our skin beyond the role it plays in aesthetics helps to reframe how we think about our skin. Having a healthy relationship with our skin is important.

What is Skin?

Skin is complex and formed of lots of different cells that exist in distinct layers in our skin ecosystem.

Each of the layers of our skin also subdivide into further layers, each with a specific function and role. Nearly all human skin is covered with hair follicles, it varies in thickness depending on where on our body it is, and it comes in a variety of skin tones.

What are the main layers of the skin?

The basic anatomy of skin is based around three main layers and they each have certain functions.

There is a lot to read and understand about the anatomy of the skin, however, below is a top-level guide to what skin is and does.

Outer layer

The epidermis is the thin outer layer of the skin. It is the only layer of skin that we see, which is why so many of us want to keep it looking in best condition. The epidermis consists of several types of cells and further sub-layers.

Squamous cells

These cells are the outermost layer, and these continuously shed, this is also known as the stratum corneum.

Basal cells

These cells are found just under the squamous cells, at the base of the epidermis.

Melanocytes

These cells are found at the base of the epidermis and make melanin. This gives our skin its colour.

Middle layer

The dermis is the middle layer of the skin. This is the layer responsible for wrinkles and where we find collagen and elastin (two proteins necessary for skin health).

The dermis has the following:

- blood vessels
- lymph vessels
- hair follicles
- sweat glands
- collagen bundles
- fibroblasts
- nerves
- sebaceous glands

The dermis is held together by collagen. This layer gives skin flexibility and strength. The dermis also has pain and touch receptors.

Deepest layer

The hypodermis is the subcutaneous fat layer, it is the deepest layer of skin and it is the reduction of tissue in this layer that causes our skin to sag as well as wrinkle.

This layer consists of a network of collagen and fat cells. It helps conserve the body's heat and protects the body from injury by acting as a shock absorber.

What is the skin barrier?

The skin barrier is a catch-all term that describes the outer layer of our skin. It has been getting a lot of attention recently as many people are having issues with their skin and lots of the causes link back to having a damaged or compromised skin barrier.

The skin barrier is also known as the stratum corneum and having a healthy skin barrier goes beyond beauty, it is about having good health.

Our skin is made up of layers, each of which perform different and essential functions in protecting our body.

The outermost layer of our skin is like a brick wall.

The best way to think about our skin barrier is that it is like a brick wall that protects us. It consists of tough skin cells that are bound together by mortar-like ceramides (lipids) that cement the skin cells together to strengthen skin. This wall is our skin barrier.

Apart from being the most visible layer of our skin, this brick wall is also hugely important in keeping us alive.

Our skin barrier is the front line of our skin, defending against damaging pollution, UV light, infection, and irritants, and locking in hydration.

The outer the layer of our skin is exposed to the world and it is the layer that we are looking after when we use skin care products. Whether through cleansing the skin, adding hydration, or locking in moisture we are nourishing our skin barrier for strength and health.

Without our skin, all sorts of harmful environmental toxins and pathogens could penetrate our skin and attack our body.

Our skin barrier is essential for good health.

Our skin is also vital for keeping water inside our bodies. Without our skin barrier, the water inside our body would escape and evaporate, leaving us completely dehydrated.

How is the skin barrier damaged?

Every day our skin faces several threats, which come from outside our body and a few that come from within.

The skin barrier defends the body against environmental threats, while simultaneously protecting our body's water balance.

The main aim of skin care is to help our skin barrier be strong.

Symptoms such as dryness, itching, and inflammation can alert us to a disturbance in this important barrier.

Environmental and intrinsic factors can upset the skin barrier and it is about having a comprehensive approach to health that can really help our skin, it is not simply about using products to fix issues.

Quite often the things we do to try and improve our skin can cause the greatest damage.

———————

There are lots of skin care products available on the market and there are now even more product launches and new hero ingredients to try.

However, all of this can get very confusing for our skin especially if we are experimenting with lots of assorted products and routines at once.

We may not always understand how harsh an ingredient is on our skin until we experience sensitivity or irritation.

Increasingly consumers are overloading their skin with lots of assorted products.

———————

Instead of protecting our skin, we end up aggravating it.

Over-cleansing and over-using products that strip the natural oils in our skin are examples of actions that can start breaking down the ceramides and lipids that help hold our skin cells together. Instead of strengthening our skin, we are damaging it through the products we use and over interference.

An area that has grown in popularity in recent years is the use of exfoliating acids. There are several types of exfoliating acids and these acids come in different strengths however, overuse of acids can also be a source of damage to our skin.

While using acids can give our face a smooth glow (when used in moderation), it is easy to get hooked on the way our skin looks after it has peeled off of old skin cells to reveal new skin and we can easily find ourselves overusing products.

Overuse of exfoliating products or use of ingredients that are too strong for our skin, has its drawbacks because it can lead to red, raw, and flaking skin and a weaker skin barrier, which brings with its other skin problems.

Finding the balance between our skin type, skin sensitivity and skin routine is key.

As well as overuse of products, some of the external and internal factors that can affect our skin barrier include:

- environments that are too humid or dry
- allergens, irritants, and pollutants
- sun exposure
- detergents and soaps

- exposure to harsh synthetic chemicals

Everyday our skin faces a range of challenges and building a skin care routine that is right for your skin type and skin condition can help keep your skin in a healthy strong condition.

What are the signs of skin barrier damage?

Skin barrier damage is increasingly common, and it is a major source of irritation to skin.

> *When our skin barrier isn't functioning properly our skin becomes compromised.*

skin can become red, irritated, shiny, sore, dry, sensitive, uncomfortable or itchy or a combination of all those things and more.

A healthy skin barrier means resilient strong and healthy-looking skin. For many years personal cosmetics tended to view skin care as something that was about preserving beauty and improving aesthetics, however increasingly we are realising that skin care is about holistic health and healthy skin.

A healthy way to approach skin care think about using products in a way that helps skin to remain strong and that may mean using fewer products, which isn't always what the beauty industry will want you to hear.

How do I protect my skin barrier?

We can help protect and repair our skin barrier by simplifying our skin care routine. This may mean using fewer products, using skin care with a suitable pH, and becoming aware of the effects of certain ingredients on our skin.

Our skin barrier is our body's defence against pathogens so keeping it healthy is much more than a cosmetic concern, here are some tips that can help.

Simplify your skin care routine

Performing a complicated daily skin routine every day that involves a lot of skincare products, can inadvertently weaken our skin barrier.

> *We need to valuate which of our skincare products are essential and effective.*

If you have a bathroom cabinet full of products, think about which ones you really need, consider why you are using that product and how your skin feels when using them.

Many of us have a shelf or a drawer that has random skincare products bought over time, some we know didn't feel right for our skin, yet it can be hard to throw them away or move on from them.

One of the areas where damage can happen unintentionally is during exfoliation. Make sure you pay attention to your skin when exfoliating, notice how your skin reacts to what you use. Avoid harsh exfoliators and over-exfoliating.

Some types of exfoliating scrubs and brushes can be too harsh for our skin and can temporarily damage our skin barrier.

In simplifying your routine, get rid of skin care products that have caused you skin irritation. Repairing a damaged skin barrier is much more time and effort than simply clearing our products that your skin gets irritated by.

Pay attention to pH

Keeping the skin's pH at a healthy level can help protect from skin conditions as the skin is naturally acidic.

The skin's acid mantle is a hugely important part of our skin.

Being aware of the role of acid and alkaline levels in our skin can help make us more aware of product impact.

Use botanical oils to replenish your skin barrier

Plant based ingredients are rich in vitamins, minerals and fatty acid and can be hugely beneficial to the skin barrier.

Not all plant oils are the same, certain plant oils can help repair and protect the skin barrier and others are simply good at preventing our skin barrier from losing water.

Many plant oils have antibacterial, anti-inflammatory, and antioxidant effects and they can be gentle and fortifying on the skin. If you want strong healthy skin, then a plant based facial oil is an essential skin protector in your skin care routine.

Formulations that include ceramides

Ceramides are waxy lipids that occur naturally in skin and they make up a large part of the skin's composition. They play a key role in protecting our skin against environmental threats.

Ceramides are found in high concentrations in the stratum corneum (the outer layer of the skin). They are important for the healthy functioning of our skin barrier and they are the glue that keep the bricks in the skin wall together.

Products containing ceramides may help improve the skin barrier and can help dryness, itchiness, and scaling caused by a poorly functioning barrier.

Not all skin care ingredients work for everyone.

No matter what the marketing messages say, the reality is that we may need to try a few products or brands to determine, which one works best for keeping your skin healthy and well moisturised.

The general advice to anyone thinking about their skin barrier health is to keep your skincare routine simple, consistent and plant based.

There are lots of products you may want to try, and innovative marketing claims are written to entice you, however skin care really does not need to be complicated.

It may be that you have some specific skin conditions, in which case treat those on a case by case basis, however day to day a less is more attitude to skincare can really help your skin.

What is the skin's acid mantle?

The skin's acid mantle is a thin film on the skin's surface including lipids from our oil glands mixed with amino acids from sweat, it is also known as the hydro lipid film. It sounds a bit grubby, but it is a natural process that is incredibly sophisticated at helping to keep us healthy.

The skin's acid mantle, along with the skin microbiome, is part of a delicate matrix that creates a healthy skin barrier. Not all the factors regulating skin surface pH are known, however, there is enough evidence to support the barrier function and the self-disinfection we get from our skin's acid mantle.

A healthy skin barrier is what gives us good skin.

The skin's acid mantle's main job is to keep the good in (such as moisture) and the bad out (such as bacteria and pollution).

An intact acid mantle biologically prevents inflammation and irritation to the skin and our approach to skin care should be about minimum disturbance of the acid mantle.

Is the acid mantle related to skin's pH?

The acid mantle is related to our skin's pH. Like many other tissues, our skin too has a specific pH, and it is on the acidic side. It is good to think about the pH of our skin as it helps us to become aware of how products and environmental factors can disrupt the balance we need for healthy skin.

It might be a long time since you were in a chemistry class however, potential Hydrogen (pH) level refers to the acidity level of substances. The pH scale measures from acid to alkaline.

The scale ranges from 1 to 14, with 7 considered "neutral" and the lower numbers are acidic, while the upper levels are alkaline.

The acid mantle gets its name from the fact that the skin's ideal pH is slightly acidic, anywhere between 4.7 and 5.75 on the pH scale.

Once we understand that our skin has an optimal acid range, we become more aware of the impact that products or our actions have on our skin which can skew our skin too alkaline (or disrupt the skin's pH level).

Every time you use a product on your skin you affect the acidic film on the skin's surface.

Finding products that are gentle to the skin is key to minimising disruption to the skin's pH level.

There are also specific products that can help re-balance the skin's pH, which is important when we think we may have disrupted our acidic balance by using a specific product (like after cleansing for example).

> *When our skin has a slightly acidic pH, the barrier is healthy and intact.*

The acidic pH of the skin protects us against overgrowth of pathogens like bacteria (that thrive at a higher more alkaline pH).

Why is skin pH important to skin health?

With more acidity on the skin, we can combat harmful microbes and damaging free radicals (that increase the ageing process and that can cause other skin irritations).

It can be challenging to level out our skin's pH, so it is much better to take care if it and be mindful of causing an imbalance.

The outer layer of our skin (the stratum corneum) can signal to the epidermis (the layer below) when our skin barrier function is disrupted, which is a remarkable activity for a dead tissue.

Rinsing skin with water alone can immediately produce a transient increase in skin pH level, which can take several hours to completely normalise, so pH awareness is a key area of consideration when it comes to your skin care routine.

What factors affect skin pH?

We can get a general idea of our skin health and pH level through observation. However, the following are all factors that can affect our skin's pH.

- Air pollution
- Cosmetics
- Detergents
- Antibacterial soaps and gels
- Sweat
- Tap water

Irritation, acne, redness, and dry spots may all be signs of a high skin pH that's leaning towards a more alkaline profile or that the acid levels have been disrupted.

When thinking about our skin's pH, we may want to think about using gentle cleansers and remember that tap water affects our skin's pH too.

There are skin care products that you can use to balance your pH levels. These are products such as toners and facial mists formulated with balancing the skin's pH in mind.

A balancing hydrating mist or skin toner can help neutralise any remaining alkalinity that's affecting our skin's optimal pH levels, particularly after cleansing.

How do I know if my acid mantle is damaged?

Dry, flaky skin, redness, sensitivity, or signs of premature ageing can all be signs that our skin's pH is out of balance and they are also signs that your skin barrier function is compromised.

Cleansing is key part of a skin care routine; however, it is also an area that has potential to disrupt the acid mantle.

Cleansers that have harsh surfactants for example, can make it challenging for the skin to hold onto its optimal pH. We may experience symptoms like stinging or dryness when using these products.

By disrupting our acid mantle through over cleansing, we can compromise our skin's ability to protect itself and retain moisture.

A destabilised skin pH also affects the skin's microbiome, which is a complex and essential population of beneficial bacteria that helps us to have healthy skin.

When our acid mantle and microbiome is out of balance, we can become susceptible to inflammatory skin conditions.

When our skin barrier is not intact, its ability to preventing allergens and irritants from entering the skin is compromised. We are more likely to have irritations, sensitivities, and skin conditions. It is vital we protect our skin barrier as so many issues stem from that barrier being compromised.

How can we protect the acid mantle?

Skin that has lost the slightly acidic coat is not only prone to dryness, itchiness, and wrinkling, it is also vulnerable to infection.

Whilst skincare products can help to support our acid mantle, it is only one part of the overall picture. Good health, a good diet (including plant oils) and exercise can give your body what it needs to support its natural acid mantle, so think of your skin are part of your overall health and wellbeing.

Here are some tips to help look after your acid mantle.

Use Fewer Products

Looking after our skin and acid mantle is often about what we should leave out of our routine than what we need to add in.

Using fewer products can be beneficial for skin.

When you consider how many complex synthetic ingredients are contained in modern skincare, the compound effect is we are layering many tens of ingredients onto our skin a day. Not all those ingredients are always good for our skin and it is also harder to find out what ingredients might be causing irritation.

Avoid harsh cleansers

Cleansers used to be about leaving skin squeaky clean, which is now being recognised as not being that good for our skin health. This approach was extremely hard on the skin, stripping out all the natural oils.

Avoid harsh cleansers or soaps that leave skin feeling tight or squeaky clean. Also avoid using abrasive loofahs or buff puffs, that feel rough against the skin. When it comes to your skin be gentle.

Skip the scrubs

It was common to find large particles in exfoliating scrubs, however these particles can be damaging to the skin. Scrubs that feel grainy or sandy should be avoided as the particles in them are large and can be too abrasive for the delicate skin on our face (and they damage the outer layer of our skin).

Limit acid exfoliation

Acid exfoliation can give impressive results however it can cause skin problems if misused or overused. You may want to limit use of acid exfoliators to once twice a week and you need to be mindful of the type and strength of acid exfoliant that you are using.

Don't use acid exfoliators without understanding what acid and strength you are using and why you are using it.

All too often we can fall into the trap of using a product that is being hyped about and we dive in and learn through trial and error, however once the skin is damaged it is much trickier to repair and calm it.

What is the skin microbiome?

Skin microbiome refers to the living protective layer on our skin. The surface of our skin is home to many complex organisms and that may sound like it is a bad thing, but they are good for you and your health.

Just like our gut, our skin is home to a community of billions of friendly living microorganisms.

These microorganisms play a vital role in our immune system and appearance.

This community of microorganisms is called skin microbiome. It is an invisible ecosystem that lives on the skin that's working all the time to help keep our skin healthy and in good condition.

Why is skin microbiome important?

Our bodies are filled with bacteria, the good and the bad. Two areas where a variety of bacteria are present are in our gut and on our skin.

The surface of the skin has its own microbiome of healthy bacteria and supporting a balance of beneficial bacteria on the skin can help the skin barrier function.

Our skin microbiome is unique to us.

Some parts of our skin microbiome are similar to others, but there are some areas that are defined by factors that are completely personal to us. These unique factors include genetics, and our lifestyle, like where we live, what we eat and even if you have pets.

Our skin microbiome is different all over our body, from our face to our underarms to our legs and our skin microbiome is a rich and diverse ecosystem.

How does the microbiome help our skin?

Our skin microbiome protects our skin from unfriendly organisms and helps manage our skin's pH.

A balanced, diverse microbiome supports many of the processes that the skin needs to stay strong and resilient.

Our microbiome makes important contributions to our skin barrier and the production of nutrients and essential skin lipids.

There are differences between the microbiome in dry, normal, oily and combination skin however, we have a lot to learn about the skin microbiome.

Skin microbiome within the beauty industry is still a new concept. It is an area that is challenging current feelings about the role of bacteria in the skin. More people are now receptive to the idea of the skin as a living ecosystem and this aligns with broader trends for more natural, holistic, and healthy beauty and skin care.

What happens when our microbiome is out of balance?

A balanced, diverse microbiome supports many of the processes that the skin needs to stay healthy and resilient.

When our microbial balance is disturbed, we may not always see a noticeable difference. But the microbiome may function less effectively, offering less support to the skin.

> *A significantly imbalanced microbiome can also affect a variety of skin conditions.*

Being aware that we have a microbiome, helps us to have an appreciation of the ecosystem that we have on the surface of our skin that keeps us healthy.

What are microbiome skin care products?

Microbiome skincare is still a new and growing area of skin care. At the moment, the main offerings in this space are focused on offering prebiotic and probiotic solutions.

If you have ever been interested in gut health, you will be familiar with probiotics in relation to gut health and cultured products. When it comes to skincare it is important to know that products have extracts made from bacteria rather than actual live cultures.

Some microbiome skincare brands take a scientific stance (with products designed to address specific concerns and benefits) while others place an emphasis on nature (overall skin health, holistic lifestyles, and green beauty).

As this category of skin care continues to grow you will notice more skin microbiome-friendly cleansers, moisturisers and skin microbiome-enhancing probiotic mists and serums available.

How does skin age?

One of the biggest areas of skincare is related to combating the signs of ageing. A lot happens to our skin as we get older and a basic understanding of the ageing process of skin helps us to understand the changes we may see in our skin as we age.

The term anti-aging in marketing messaging, can suggests that ageing is somehow an undesirable thing, however ageing is not something we should feel awkward about.

Ageing skin cannot be reversed with products yet our skin care routine and the products we use can influence the appearance of these changes, to keep skin healthy looking.

HEALTHY SKIN x HEALTHY VIBES

As we grow older our skin cell turnover starts to gradually slow down and continues to decline as we age.

———————

Alongside the natural aging process are several external factors that can produce added ageing effects and they are the ones that we have the most influence over (such as changes to lifestyle and having a good skin care routine).

As skin ages it experiences a slowing down of its natural processes, which impact skin firmness, tautness, and brightness. The causes of biological ageing are uncertain and there are several reasons related to why our organisms deteriorate as we grow older.

Visible signs of skin ageing (spots, fine lines, wrinkles) may appear because of our skin's natural defence mechanisms, as well as slower cell renewal, cell turnover, activity, and recovery.

Our skin is constantly ageing, but we tend not to think of it as ageing until it starts to show.

———————

What causes these visible signs of ageing is complex and varies according to our genetics and our lifestyle and environment.

As we grow older, lots of different processes and hormonal changes take place in the skin that change its appearance, structure and even how it feels.

What is happening to skin in our twenties?

As early as in our twenties unhealthy lifestyle habits, environmental damage and UV exposure can start to change our skin.

Our cell defences may begin to weaken against free radicals, and our natural ability to fight off skin damage declines. Cell renewal and turnover rates also naturally start to slow, diminishing skin radiance.

What is happening to skin in our thirties?

In our 30s, collagen (which keeps skin firm) and elastin (which keeps skin bouncing back) begin to degrade, which may result in the start of visible wrinkles.

Cell renewal and turnover continue to decline, leading to a duller complexion and uneven skin tone.

What is happening to skin in our forties?

By our forties, skin appears thinner and its naturally protective barrier lipids are not as pronounced. Depending on hormonal activity, we may experience uneven skin tone to adult acne.

More prominent signs of skin ageing can also appear, such as dark spots and significant dullness.

What is happening to skin in our fifties onward?

The lipids in our skin barrier reduce leading to less efficient moisture retention (and more potential for sensitivity and dehydration). By now, skin can show prominent wrinkles, fine lines, and discoloration.

> *One of the biggest changes to skin can happen during menopause.*

During the menopause, your body stops making as much collagen. This can cause a loss of fat under the skin and the skin's elasticity drops. Skin also becomes thinner in menopause, since there's a relationship between collagen production, skin thickness, and lack of oestrogen (a hormone).

As the natural lipids in our skin diminish, skin can experience greater sensitivity and after the age of 50, there is evidence to suggest that the pH level of our skin gets higher. It becomes important in these years to repair the skin's moisture barrier with good, effective skin care.

Does the skin renew itself?

You may have wondered why brands say you need to try a skincare product for at least twenty-eight days before you see results. This is because of how our skin renews itself.

Our skin is constantly shedding, and this is part of a healthy skin cycle.

―――――――――

Our skin is constantly making way for new skin cells, which are being formed in the deepest layer of the epidermis.

New cells work their way up to the surface of the skin and the skin cell on the top layer will flake off (either on its own or with help from an exfoliator).

A skin cycle can vary with each individual and factors such as our age, hormones, skin condition and health can impact the average cycle but on average our skin regenerates itself approximately every twenty-eight days in our twenties (however cell turn over can take longer as we age).

In middle age it can take between twenty-eight and forty-two days and from our fifties onwards it can be significantly longer.

Skin renewal happens because of skin cells travelling from the lowest epidermis layer of the skin to the top layer.

―――――――――

The longer cell renewal takes, the larger the build-up of dead skin on the surface, which can leave skin looking dull. Regular gentle exfoliating as part of a skincare routine is therefore essential to help slough away the build-up.

What are skin types?

Understanding our skin type can help us understand the skin we have and the kinds of skin care products we may need to help keep our skin healthy. Skin type categorises some key characteristics of skin into broad groups.

It is a good idea to think about what kind of skin type you have as it will help shape your skin care choices.

Skin type should not be confused with skin conditions. Skin conditions are temporary states which may change over the course of your lifetime, while your skin type is more about the kind of skin you are born with. There are four basic types of skin:

- Normal
- Dry
- Oily
- Combination

As well as taking a closer look at our own skin, we may want to think about the skin type that runs in our family.

Skin type is determined by genetics.

Even though skin type is determined by our genes, it is important to note that the condition of our skin can vary according to what is going on in our lives, including the internal and external factors that our skin is exposed to. Skin conditions are not always something that can be dealt with in isolation.

What is my skin type?

You may know what your skin type is from observation, however for others it can be hard to assess especially if you are dealing with any skin conditions as well.

What is normal skin?

Calling anything normal feels a bit unfair, however, normal skin often has no major concerns.

If you have fine pores, an even complexion with a good balance of oils, means this skin type is likely to be normal skin. It is also a sign that your skincare routine is working well for your skin's needs.

What is dry skin?

Dry skin is lacking in natural oils that our skin produces. Our skin may look and feel dry, dull, and flaky and feels like it lacks moisture and lipids.

Dry skin is less elastic and may feel tighter and it can feel itchy or even sore. Dry skin is particularly susceptible to environmental influences, such as sunlight or wind.

What is combination skin?

Combination skin tends to have two skin types across the face, and it is one of the most common skin types.

It may be normal to dry skin around the cheeks and chin and oily and blemished skin around the T-zone of the forehead and nose.

What is oily skin?

An oily skin type has excess oil on the face which may produce a persistently shiny or greasy appearance.

Oily skin has a tendency for pores to become clogged and enlarged and dead skin cells may accumulate. Blackheads, pimples, and other types of acne are also common with this skin type.

What are skin conditions?

There are many kinds of skin conditions, these may be temporary or long-term problems and we may experience a range of them over time. Below are some of the most common.

Sensitive Skin

Sensitive skin can easily be irritated and may react to certain products with redness, burning, or itching.

With sensitive skin, proper and gentle skin care is important.

While many people can have a skin reaction at some point or another to a product or ingredient, those with persistent issues are classified as having sensitive skin, below are some of the signs of sensitive skin.

Skin easily flushes
Redness is a common sign of sensitive skin, whether it is genetic or a reaction to certain ingredients. Those with truly sensitive skin have this reaction often.

Prone to rashes and bumps
Frequent rashes and tiny red bumps are a sign of sensitivity.

Products sting or burn
People with sensitive skin tend to have a thinner skin barrier, allowing the ingredients in skin care products to sting or burn. Don't overload sensitive skin with harsh ingredients. Stick with gentle, natural products.

Dry patches
Dryness and irritation of the skin may be signs of eczema, a type of dermatitis characterised by a leaky skin barrier that doesn't effectively trap moisture. Scaling and flaking develop the longer the dryness persists.

Itchy skin
Itchy, taut skin is a symptom of sensitive skin which can be easily worsened by washing with hot water. Switch to a lukewarm water and avoid hot water in your routine.

Broken Capillaries
Broken capillaries are tiny blood vessels that become visible near the surface of the skin and are often seen on the nose and cheeks. Those with sensitive skin, which is thin and has fewer protective layers—are more prone to having visible broken capillaries.

Fragrance is an issue
Scented products are a common trigger for those with sensitive skin and they can quickly inflame the skin.

Dehydrated Skin

Dehydrated skin is a common skin condition, caused by a loss of water in the skin. Dehydrated skin may feel tight and look dull.

Dehydrated skin can appear dry, but it is different from having a dry skin type. While dehydrated skin lacks water, dry skin lacks natural oils.

Any skin type can become dehydrated including dry, normal, and even oily skin. Dry and dehydrated skin may sometime feel similar.

Acne

Acne is a common skin problem among teenagers, but it can also affect adults well into their thirties and beyond.

Adult acne is also becoming increasingly common. It is unclear why this is happening (however a combination of stress, dietary factors and changing hormones may be contributing to its rise).

Like the acne we may get as a teenager, adult acne is a skin condition that occurs when your hair follicles become plugged with oil and dead skin cells.

The pattern of adult acne may be different to that in teens. In teens, it is often found on the forehead and cheeks, but in adults you can see it more often on the lower face along the jawline.

Women are more likely to have adult acne than men. It is thought that many cases of adult acne are caused by changes in hormone levels that many women have from periods, pregnancy, and polycystic ovary syndrome.

> **Treatment for acne depends on how severe it is, and it can take months of treatment before symptoms improve.**

Rosacea

Rosacea is a condition that seems to be on the increase. It is a long-term skin condition that affects the face.

It is more common in women and people with lighter skin. The signs of rosacea include a redness (blushing) across your nose, cheeks, forehead, and chin that comes and goes.

You may also feel a burning or stinging feeling when using water or skincare products.

As rosacea gets worse, your cheeks, nose, skin, and forehead can appear red most of the time and you may get small pink or red bumps. Sometimes these become filled with a yellowish liquid.

> **It is not clear what causes rosacea, however some triggers can make symptoms worse.**

Alcohol, spicy foods, cheese, and caffeine as examples of rosacea triggers.

There are no cures for rosacea but treatment from a GP can help control the symptoms.

Blemished Skin

There are many types of skin blemishes, but they are areas of uneven skin, differently coloured skin tone, dry patches or oiliness, found typically on the face. There are several reasons why we might have blemishes on our skin, and it is more of a catch-all term (covering anything from skin blemishes cause by hormonal changes, scaring, blackheads, and whiteheads to form).

The causes of blemishes could be down to genetics, stress, or hormonal fluctuations.

Hyperpigmentation

Hyperpigmentation can show on the skin as small, dark patches. It appears when your skin produces too much melanin (because of exposure to UV rays from the sun). There are also other factors which can cause hyperpigmentation, including hormonal changes such as during pregnancy, acne scars, as well as certain illnesses.

Other Skin Conditions

There are many other skin conditions that can affect the skin that may need more specific attention.

Examples of these include:

- Dermatitis - a general term for inflammation of the skin. Atopic dermatitis (a type of eczema) is the most common form.

- Eczema - can cause the skin to become itchy, dry, cracked, and sore (the exact cause may not be down to one single thing).

- Psoriasis - can cause a variety of skin rashes including silver scales on the skin. People with psoriasis have an increased production of skin cells. Although the process is not fully understood, it's thought to be related to a problem with the immune system.

There are several types of skin conditions and causes for them and the above list is not exhaustive.

What causes dark eye circles?

There are several factors for dark circles under the eyes. Whilst an eye serum may be able to help brighten the area, not all of them can help, as the reason for dark circles under the eyes can be due to a variety of reasons. Dark circles are also more common in people with darker skin tones. Some common causes for dark circles include:

Genetics

Family history plays a part in whether we have dark circles under our eyes. A family tendency to have dark circles around the eyes or just under the eye area may be an inherited condition.

Fatigue

Tiredness can cause dark circles to appear more visible because of our skin becoming dull and pale (allowing for dark tissues and blood vessels beneath our skin to show).

Age

As we get older, our skin becomes thinner. We also lose the fat and collagen needed to keep our skin's elasticity. As this occurs, the dark blood vessels beneath our skin become more visible.

Dehydration

Dehydration is also a cause of dark circles under our eyes. When our body is dehydrated, the skin beneath our eyes begins to look dull and our eyes look sunken.

Sun overexposure

Over exposure to the sun can cause our body to produce an excess of melanin (the pigment that provides our skin with colour). This can lead to excess pigmentation showing through the thin skin underneath the eyes.

How does the sun affect skin?

Sunlight, in moderation, is good for our skin but overexposure to the sun can damage skin both on the surface and at a cellular level.

There are different rays that make up sunlight and they have positive and negative effects on skin condition and can influence the way our skin reacts to the sun.

Some light can be detected by the human eye, while other light (such as ultraviolet light and infrared light) is not visible to the human eye.

Too much sun causes skin damage. Premature skin ageing is one of the most common, when skin ages prematurely and starts to sag and develop wrinkles before its time.

A majority of premature skin ageing is thought to be caused by the sun and is known as photoaging.

The direct DNA damage caused by UVB rays plays a role in photoaging, but the main cause is the oxidative stress triggered by sunlight rays.

Free radicals caused by sun exposure induce not only stressed skin cells they also break down collagen and elastin which are important for smooth, plumped skin.

How does the sun cause oxidative stress?

Certain light rays interact with skin cells and generate free radicals. These free radicals are highly reactive oxygen molecules, and the body uses antioxidants to neutralise them.

When there is an imbalance between the production of free radicals and the body's ability to neutralise them, the free radicals start to damage cells in a process known as oxidative stress.

Oxidative stress is a big contributor in our skins ageing process and it contributes to the loss of collagen resulting in fine lines. Oxidative stress is also involved in reduced barrier function, decreased moisture, and increased skin cancer risk (due to DNA mutations).

Why do we get wrinkles?

Wrinkles are the lines and creases that form in our skin and they are a natural part of ageing (and are most prominent on sun-exposed skin).

Some wrinkles can become deep crevices or furrows and may be especially noticeable around our eyes, mouth, and neck.

Genetics play a large part in determining our skin's structure and texture.

———————

As we age fat in the deeper layers of our skin diminishes as we age. This causes loose, saggy skin and more pronounced lines and crevices.

Pollutants and smoking also contribute to wrinkling as we get older, our skin naturally becomes less elastic and more fragile.

Decreased production of natural oils dries our skin and makes it appear more wrinkled.

———————

Facial movements and expressions, such as squinting or smiling, can also lead to fine lines and wrinkles.

Does skin differ between gender?

The components and structure of men and women's skin are the same there are hormonal differences.

Testosterone levels in men contribute to thicker skin in men and beard growth the most visible difference between the facial skin of men and women.

The outer layer of the skin is slightly thicker in men and coupled with the increase in active hair follicles, this contributes to a significantly rougher facial texture.

Regular shaving can also make male skin more stressed and skin can become more sensitive and react faster.

A lot of men have shaving-related skin problems.

Daily shaving stresses the skin and can cause irritation. It removes the uppermost layer of skin cells, exposing immature skin that is particularly sensitive to external influences.

Do men and women need to use different skincare products?

Although there are a lot of gender specific skincare brands, men and women do not materially need to use different skincare products.

Men and women's skin are structurally quite similar and both can benefit from a skin care routine.

A routine that includes gentle cleansing, hydration, moisture, and SPF is good for skin regardless of gender.

A lot of what the beauty industry has done historically with regards to men and women's skincare is marketing. There may be skin concerns that need specific attention and care should be given to select skincare product that help the skin based on concerns (rather than based on gender).

2 Skin Care

There are benefits to having a simple skincare routine and looking after your skin does not need to be complicated.

The main thing with skin care is consistency and using fewer and kinder ingredients on your skin.

It is also important to remember that to have healthy skin, you need a healthy lifestyle, so diet, sleep, stress, and our overall wellness can all affect our skin. Cosmetic products alone cannot fix underlying health issues that affect your skin.

What are the benefits of having a skin care routine?

Whatever your skin type, a regular routine can help keep your skin healthy and happy. It doesn't take long either, just five minutes a day can make a difference.

There are several benefits of a daily skin care routine and supporting one can help to fortify your skin and keep it looking in good condition.

> *A skincare routine can help improve the health of our skin and it can help us feel better too.*

When we take care of our skin regularly and appropriately it will be healthier, and it can help support a good strong skin barrier.

As well as having healthy skin, here are some of the reasons you might want to get into the habit of looking after your skin.

Helps slow down ageing

While in our twenties and early thirties we may not have to worry much about the signs of visible ageing, having a daily skincare routine can help to slow down the effects of ageing in the long term.

> *As we grow older, our skin begins to lose its strength and elasticity.*

When we cleanse, exfoliate, moisturise, and use sunscreen on a regular basis, we fortify our skin and give our skin some of its strength and elasticity back in the process (which helps our skin as we age).

Boosts confidence

When we take care of our skin, we may also be helping to beat our insecurities. Healthy strong skin can make us feel good.

The routine of cleansing our face or massaging on a facial oil, not only makes our skin feel better, it can make us feel better.

The feeling of healthy skin is a great confidence boost

Skincare as self-care

After a long or stressful day, self-care in the form of a skincare routine can an effective way to relax or unwind.

A skincare routine can help our stress levels and our skin.

Using a nourishing face mask or taking the time for ourselves to use skin products can help us to reduce our stress levels and it can have lots of benefits to our skin

How do I build a skincare routine?

When it comes to building a skin care routine, simplicity and consistency are key. To protect and fortify your skin, minimising the steps can help decrease your chances of skin irritation.

Some skin care routines have ten steps, but this is not entirely necessary for the skin.

There are many downfalls to having a multi-step, product heavy daily routine (including redness and sensitivity).

Skin sensitivity due to extensive routines is a valid concern especially with so many products available on the market, consumers are mixing product combinations and then find that they end up with flared, irritated skin.

An effective routine can be created in very few steps. It does not need to be complicated.

Simple skin care routine

1. Cleanse
2. Hydrating Mist
3. Moisturise
4. SPF (day)

You may prefer a routine with more stages and products; however, a simple minimal routine can be highly effective in protecting our skin barrier.

What is cleansing?

There has been a lot of focus on cleansing in recent years. This is because cleansing is an essential part of any skincare routine.

Cleansing our skin helps remove dirt, oil, pollution, and other unwanted debris from our skin. It is key to helping keep our skin in good condition. It is not a step that you should cut corners on.

Throughout the day the skin on is continually covered with bacteria, pollutants, viruses, dirt, and dead skin cells.

Cleansing is the part of our routine that help remove this surface build up and allow a clean base for other skincare products that follow.

How do I cleanse?

There are lots of types of cleansers, however you should look for one that is gentle and suitable for your skin type. Plant oil-based balm cleansers are kind to the skin however there are many cleansers you might want to explore (such as gel cleansers, foam cleansers, cleansing oils, lotions, and creams).

Depending on the state of your skin, cleansing your face once may be enough (usually a single cleanse in the morning for example may be all you need). Others like to cleanse their skin twice and this is known as double cleansing.

For the first cleanse, use a natural cleansing balm or oil.

To cleanse well you need to get comfortable with massaging the cleanser around your face. This is a good chance to lift dirt from your skin and give yourself a bit of a face massage.

Cleansing with an oil-based cleanser is not a quick job, it requires effort help loosen the debris on the skin. You don't need to be rough, but you do need to be patient.

Massaging the cleanser into your skin will allow enough time for a thorough cleanse, really working the cleanser and ingredients into the skin. You can also use cleaning as a time to give your face a little bit of a facial massage.

Try not to be too harsh with the movements, avoid hard scrubbing or rubbing.

To remove the cleanser, use a clean cotton cloth or flannel that has been warmed under a hot tap.

Use the cloth to swipe clean and remove the cleanser, making sure you cover your whole face and rinse the cloth as you go along.

Water temperature matters when it comes to skincare as hot water can strip our skin of its natural oils.

At this point you either move to the next step of our routine or to do a second cleanse (particularly if you have been exposed to pollution, dust or are wearing heavy make-up that day).

For the second cleanse use wet fingers to work the cleanser more deeply into the skin using small circular motions with our fingertips.

Work around the nose, chin area and hairline.

Remove the cleanser using the warm cloth method.

How does cleansing help other products?

Cleansing is an effective way to prepare our skin for other skincare products.

Congested pores can not only cause breakouts but also prevent the absorption of other skincare products. Cleansing daily will help to clear our pores and ensure that the active ingredients in our moisturisers and serums can penetrate the deeper layers of the skin.

Why we need a hydrating mist?

Face mists are quite an underappreciated product in the world of skincare, however they are gaining popularity. Face mists are refreshing, hydrating and can help keep moisture. They increasingly come with a range of added benefits including prebiotics, antioxidants, and pH balancing ingredients.

A good face mist can help fight dryness and brighten dull complexions.

A gentle botanical face mist also will work with every skin type.

A good face mist will include ingredients that promote hydration and water retention.

Look for mists that have ingredients such as hyaluronic acid and glycerin. These ingredients help hydration and help to hold in moisture and heal the damaged skin barrier.

A face mist can also that have antioxidants or fermented fruit extracts that help skin combat the effects of free radicals and daily exposure to pollutants in city life.

> *Rose water mists can be effective in reducing inflammation and soothing acne-prone skin.*

Always check the ingredients labels and look for an alcohol-free mist as alcohol dries out the skin's surface.

A facial mist should be used after cleansing twice daily; however, you can mist more often during the day, (especially if you are traveling, in a heated room, feeling hot and flushed or your skin needs a pick-me-up).

What are the benefits of exfoliation?

Exfoliation is the removal of the dead skin cells on the skin's surface.

> *Exfoliating helps keep our skin smooth and healthy.*

As we age, our cell regeneration slows down, which means our skin is slower to shed skin cells and generate new ones.

When old skin cells start to build up on the surface of our skin, it can leave our faces looking dull, rough, or dry. A build-up of dead skin cells can also result in excess oil and clogged pores.

Exfoliation helps remove the barrier of dead skin cells clogging the skin and uncovers fresh new cells below.

This not only makes our skin look brighter, it also offers a skin surface that allow other products to penetrate more deeply into the skin, which makes them more effective.

A regular exfoliating routine can help you have healthy fresh skin however, it is important to make sure exfoliation is gentle.

Over exfoliation can be harmful for our skin barrier.

You can build in exfoliation as part of your skincare routine and for most twice a week is enough.

Allowing dead cells to build up on the skin can leave skin feeling tight, dry, and flaky. Regular exfoliation helps remove dead skin to smooth the skin's texture.

Regular exfoliation helps to clear pores and prevent acne build up. As well as dislodging dirt and grime, it removes dead skin cells which can block the pores and lead to acne.

Exfoliation also has anti-ageing benefits. By removing the top layer of dead skin cells and revealing the new cells underneath, we can prompt new cell turnover to keep the skin bright. This becomes more important as the skin matures and renews itself less often.

Exfoliation also helps other skincare work harder. Dead skin can act as a barrier, preventing other skincare from penetrating the epidermis as effectively. By gently buffing away these dead cells, our skin can better absorb moisture, hydration, and other targeted skincare products.

What is difference between chemical and physical exfoliants?

Physical exfoliation is when you manually remove dead skin. It can be cleansing brush or an exfoliating skincare product with tiny particles in such as silica, sugar, or ground fruit seeds.

Chemical exfoliants are acids or enzymes that get rid of dead skin cells.

Chemical exfoliants come in various concentrations and work by breaking down the proteins that bind the skin cells in the top layer of our skin.

Chemical exfoliation does not require scrubbing or physical abrasion and they can be gentler on our skin, if used in a low percentage.

Why do we need to hydrate?

Dehydrated skin is a skin condition, and it means that our skin is lacking water.

Any skin type can become dehydrated including dry, normal, and even oily skin.

ZAFFRIN O'SULLIVAN

Dehydration means that our body is losing more water than it is taking in.

Water is especially important to our overall health. Like any other organ in your body, your skin's tissue is made up of many kinds of cells, which all need the right amount of water to function properly.

The skin performs many essential functions but most importantly it is a protective barrier to keep harmful things like micro-organisms from entering our bodies. Skin that is not hydrated enough will become dry, tight, and flaky.

Dehydrated skin is less resilient and small gaps can open between the cells in the outer layers of the skin, making the skin barrier less robust at keeping harmful things out of the skin.

You can help your skin to remain healthy and well hydrated by consuming enough water from the food and drink in your diet.

Whilst drinking plenty of water is still the easiest way to hydrate your skin, those with dehydrated skin may want to supplement with a topical hydrator like a face mist that binds and draws water into the cells.

Humectants such as glycerin help our skin to improve its ability to hydrate itself over time so look for them in your ingredients list.

Hydrating mists are appropriate for all skin types.

What is the difference between moisturising and hydrating?

Moisturising and hydrating both address helping made make sure the skin is getting all the water it needs to fight dryness and dehydration.

The difference, between hydrating and moisturising is that hydration is about the water content within the cells and moisturising is about trapping and sealing in moisture to build the skin's protective barrier.

Moisturisers help prevent water loss from the skin and keep the skin soft and smooth.

Does the order of applying skincare products matter?

Applying our skin care products in the proper order ensures our skin receives the full benefits of each product.

The order of product application is important.

The skin's job is to keep things out, but many of the skin care products we use have ingredients we want to get in.

Only a small amount of these key ingredients can penetrate the skin, even when perfectly formulated and applied.

If we do not apply products in the correct order, we will not always see the best results from our skin care routine or get the best from the products we use.

What is a basic morning routine?

The morning routine is all about protection from the sun, pollution, and the elements.

Morning Cleanse

In the morning, cleansing our face is beneficial because it helps to remove toxins, dead skin cells and excess oils the skin secretes overnight.

A gentle cleanser can also help to balance our skin and supply a fresh surface for the start of the day allowing for better penetration of skincare products and makeup.

Hydrating Mist

Follow your cleanse with a face mist to hydrate the skin. This will help add moisture and help return the skin's pH after cleansing. Spray mist evenly around your face.

Look for hydrating mists that are infused with different active ingredients and that have a humectant like glycerin.

Eye Serum

Apply your eye serum before applying your wider face products. This step is about supporting the health and strength of the skin under the eyes. Improving the skin quality in this area early on helps to improve appearance later.

Serum/Oil

Serums and botanical face oils are nutrient-dense treatments so keep them as close to the skin as possible.

There are various serums and face oils available but for daytime, recommended is an antioxidant serum or oil, which provide a variety of benefits helping protect our skin barrier against environmental pollutants.

Sunscreen

SPF should be the last step in your daytime skin care routine.

What is a basic evening routine?

Our skin naturally repairs itself at night and our evening time routine is all about treatment and giving our skin what it needs to re-charge.

If our skin is looking dull, now is the time to exfoliate. If it is irritated, then now is the time to hydrate and protect.

Evening Cleanse

In the evening, it is important to remove make up, dirt and debris that our skin will have collected throughout the day.

As with the morning, freshly cleansed skin allows for better penetration of any skincare products that we use on our skin in the evening.

Remove dirt, oil and makeup with an oil cleanser or cleansing balm to help dissolve and cleanse the skin.

Exfoliate

If you use an exfoliator now is the time to use it.

Some skincare routines may recommend exfoliating at least once a day, however specific exfoliating once or twice a week is enough.

Over exfoliation can lead to skin sensitivities, so be careful not to use products that are too harsh for your skin.

———————

You may be able to incorporate exfoliating enzymes into your routine by way of your facial mist, which can act as a micro-exfoliator and is gentle for use every day.

Exfoliation tackles cellular build up and reduces skin dullness.

———————

Avoid scrubs that buff away dead skin as they are often too abrasive for the skin.

Mask

The best time to put on a face mask is after cleansing or exfoliating. Using a face mask without cleansing first will trap all the day's grime underneath it.

Using a face mask any later in your routine will remove the benefit of your facial mists and serums.

Do not overuse face masks, one or two times a week is enough, to not irritate the skin.

Hydrating Mist

Apply your face mist after cleansing, as you do as part of the morning routine.

Eye Serum

As in the morning, apply your eye serum before applying your wider face products. If you wish to use an eye serum only once a day, the evening routine is the better routine to opt for.

Serum/ Face Oil

Some people use the same serum or facial oil for day and night.

Night products can be thicker and heavier as they can be absorbed over the course of several hours.

Facial oils and serums used at night create a protective coating on the skin to prevent water evaporation while we sleep.

Maintaining a high water content in the skin is key for healing and supporting healthy skin.

A facial oil or oil serum should be our last step because of the barrier that it creates on top of the skin.

Keep your skincare routine simple.
———

Adapt and adjust your skincare routine according to your needs. We are all unique and nobody else has our skin. It is important we find what works for each of us and to always be kind to our skin.

What is a facial oil?

A facial oil is an oil-based formula that is used keep the layers of our skin soft, seal in hydration and protect against allergens and pathogens (by keeping the stratum corneum intact).

Oil in our skin helps prevent water from escaping from our skin and that keeps skin hydrated.

> *Using a facial oil will help supplement natural oils, add moisture, and help repair the skin barrier.*

The biggest benefit that comes with an oil is the moisturising benefit and botanical oils that are made from plant ingredients (like pressed ingredients from seeds and nuts) are the best.

Our skin naturally produces various oils and lipids, which are used to keep our skin hydrated by preventing water loss.

Face oils complement and work alongside the natural oils in our skin.

You may be wondering if you still need to use a moisturiser alongside a face oil and the answer depends on your routine.

If you are using a hydrating mist as part of your skincare routine, then locking in water with a facial oil will help ensure skin remains hydrated and nourished for longer.

Face oils are made purely from oils, while moisturisers tend to be made from oils and water and as a result moisturisers tend to come with many other ingredients, to help the oil and water to mix together properly.

Plant oils are compatible with our skin and can help nourish the skin's top layer, which is important for our skin barrier health.

Water based products like moisturisers are important for our skin too. Whilst they still provide a small amount of oil to help the skin's barrier function, the main priority of these is to provide hydration, and this is often from water-soluble active ingredients.

When to use a face mask?

Regardless of your skin type you may want to consider using a face mask as part of your skincare routine. Face masks come in lots of different varieties such as clay masks, gel masks, exfoliating masks to hydrating overnight masks and they can be used for various kinds of skin benefits according to your needs.

You may want to incorporate a face mask into your routine, and this is best done in the evening after cleansing your skin.

It is important to make sure you do not apply your face mask to unclean skin.

Depending on the type of mask you choose, masking is not something you need to do every day. For most, a face mask used once or twice a week to compliment your daily skincare routine can offer your skin enhanced benefits (and is also a wonderful way to relax).

What are the benefits of using a clay mask?

Clay has been used on skin for thousands of years and it has lots of benefits for skin. It is suitable for most skin types. Rose clay is abundant in rich minerals and can help to replenish and restore the skin.

Clay face masks can help improve the skin in several ways. Clay can help deep cleanse skin, by drawing out impurities from the pores, Clay can help absorb excess oil from the skin, which means it is effective at helping remove extra sebum from the skin. Clay masks can also be relaxing and a natural skin soother.

Why you should avoid sheet masks?

Sheet masks have become quite popular recently however, the merits of using them aside, one of the reasons you may want to consider side-stepping them is because of the environmental impact.

> *Sheet masks like makeup wipes create a lot of unnecessary rubbish.*

Every sheet mask comes in a single use pouch and the mask inside may even be wrapped in plastic. Sheet mask pouches are made from a combination of materials such as aluminium and plastic, which are also difficult to recycle.

Sheet masks are often made of a blend of synthetic materials such as nylon, plastic microfibers and polyester which do not easily decompose when thrown away. In addition, sheet masks often include synthetic ingredients that can bio-accumulate. If you have a choice, give sheet masks a swerve.

What is retinol?

Retinol is also known as vitamin A and it is an anti-aging ingredient. It is used for reducing the appearance of wrinkles, refining skin texture and improving uneven skin tone.

Retinols come in different strengths and in various types of product. They work by speeding up cell turnover and exfoliating older cells at an increased rate (which increases elastin and collagen production).

Retinol works on a cellular level and not just a topical level, which means some are only available with a prescription.

Why you need an SPF?

SPF means 'sun protection factor'. SPF designations are only required to protect us from UVB rays. However, UVA rays are also damaging. It's important to check that your sun cream protects from both UVB and UVA rays. UVA ray protection is typically indicated by an additional tiered star system.

Wear an SPF even when the sun is not shining. UV rays can affect our skin all year, so even in winter.

The sun is the most significant cause of ageing skin.

UV rays pass through windows and are even harmful to our skin on cloudy, misty, and rainy days.

We are only partially protected when we sit in the shade or wear a sun hat. Surfaces such as water, sand, concrete, grass, snow, and ice reflect the sunlight onto our skin, giving we an even larger dose of the sun's rays. So, protect your skin from UV rays every day.

How does trans-epidermal water loss (TEWL) effect skin?

Trans-epidermal water loss (you may see it written as TEWL for short) describes a situation when the water in our skin passes from the dermis through the epidermis and evaporates from the skin's surface. It is a type of water loss that passes up through the deeper layers of our skin through to the top.

When water evaporates from our skin faster than it is replaced, skin becomes dehydrated.

This can lead to rough, itchy, or irritated skin that can appear more aged, as fine lines and wrinkles are accentuated.

Trans-epidermal water loss is a natural process in the skin however, certain things, such as the weather, the season, UV light, low-humidity and harsh skin care products can all impact trans-epidermal water loss in our skin.

One of the main functions of our skincare is to prevent water loss from our skin and moisturising is key to this.

How to treat dehydrated skin?

Dehydration is treatable with lifestyle changes. Replenishing our hydration is key, so it is important to drink plenty of water.

To keep healthy looking skin here are some straightforward ways to stay hydrated.

- Drink water throughout the day to keep skin hydrated. It also gets rid of waste and toxins in our body, which are causes of dull skin.

- Make sure you are getting enough water, especially if you think you might be exposed to common dehydration culprits like alcohol, caffeine, salty foods, and tobacco.

- Incorporating a hydrating mist into our routine (usually after cleansing) can be highly effective.

- Make sure your hydrating mist has a humectant like glycerin.

- Follow your mist with a facial oil as the lipids will help seal the hydration and create a healthy balance within the skin.

- Reduce the temperature

- Hot baths and showers can dry our skin out by breaking down the lipid barrier in our skin. This makes it easier for our skin to lose its moisture. Use lukewarm water to prevent parched skin.

Why does skin feel different in winter?

During the colder months, the main factors contributing to our skin feeling different are temperature, heating, and sunshine.

Cold Weather

During the winter, the cold and wind can reduce the moisture levels in our skin.

Reduced moisture in our skin can make our skin dry, rough, or tight, and it may feel more sensitive.

Dry skin is particularly common on the face during winter because it's more exposed to the weather.

Indoor Heat

In the winter, it is not only the cold weather that can affect our skin's condition

Central heating is also responsible for drying out the air. This adds to the water loss in our skin, which can leave we with dehydrated skin.

When our skin begins to lose its moisture and becomes dehydrated, it means it lacks the water levels needed to function effectively.

Less Sunshine

With less sunshine in the darker winter months, our skin is also losing access to nutrients, like Vitamin D, which can cause the skin to look dull.

It's essential to continue our skincare routine in winter and to use gentle products and ingredients that won't strip away our skin's natural moisture barrier.

What is maskne?

Maskne is a term that covers skin irritation and acne that can come because of wearing a face mask or other protective face covering. Face coverings and face masks can cause a mixture of uncomfortable issues for our skin.

Some of the common problems include:

- rashes from the friction of the face mask chafing against skin

- acne that has been aggravated by face coverings touching the skin

- flare ups of eczema and psoriasis

- irritation and sores from poorly made face masks or rough materials

- blocked pores and accumulations of sweat.

How to keep skin healthy while wearing a face mask?

If wearing a face mask or face covering is affecting your skin, here are some tips for what you can do to keep your skin strong and healthy.

Cotton Face Mask over synthetic fabric

Try to choose a face mask made of natural materials like cotton. Cotton will feel more breathable on the skin, whilst synthetic fabrics keep more heat and moisture and make skin feel congested.

Wash your face mask regularly

Cloth face masks should be washed regularly. Over time your face mask fabric will absorb your skin's natural oils as well as accumulating bacteria, which could lead to breakouts on your skin.

Use a plant oil or serum to protect skin

Protecting the skin barrier is key when wearing a face mask. This means fortifying the skin by using a facial oil or serum before putting on your face mask or face covering.

Using a facial oil can help protect areas of your skin from friction or chafing. Plant based ingredients are preferable as they are more readily matched to the oils in your skin. Plant oils are highly moisturising and help fortify the lipid barrier in your skin. Healthy and strong skin will be more resilient to the effects of a face mask.

Stay hydrated

Wearing a face mask means that we may find we drink less during the day due to our faces being covered. It is important to make sure you are hydrated, as this will improve the barrier function of your skin as part of your overall skin health.

Cleansing is key

Cleansing and nourishing the skin daily will ensure good skin barrier maintenance and repair. Cleansing removes natural debris and pollution that may have built up under your face mask or face covering, make sure you use a gentle cleanser and pat dry your skin.

Avoid harsh exfoliants

If your skin is irritated from wearing a face mask avoid harsh scrubs or chemical exfoliators that may worsen the problem.

Wear less make-up

Face masks create a humid environment that can lead to clogged pores and breakouts, so wear less makeup to prevent clogging of pores under the mask. If you must wear make-up above the face mask is best and now is the time to think about using an eye serum.

Invest in a face mist

Use a botanical face mist after wearing a face mask to hydrate and refresh your face, refine the surface of the skin and rebalance your skin's pH levels. This will help to prevent pores from becoming clogged.

Use a face mask treatment

At the end of a week, it is good to use a gentle face mask to cleanse and purge the skin as part of your overall skincare. Botanical ingredients are soothing and can help calm your skin as part of your routine.

3 The Beauty Industry

In recent years consumers have become more interested in how their cosmetic products are made. From the food we eat to the clothes we wear, we are asking more questions about the materials used, where they came from and at what cost to people and planet.

However, the beauty industry is hard to navigate when it comes to answering some of these questions.

How much do you know about how your skincare products are made?

Skincare products that you see in large retailers are often produced in bulk at an industrial scale. In recent years there has also been a growing interest in small batch skincare and there are multiple artisan skincare producers working in this area.

Manufacturing skin care products whether at a small scale or a large scale requires a lot of consideration to shelf life, ingredients, and preservatives, to keep the texture intact and the products fresh.

A few major multinational companies run the beauty industry. They own and service an entire range of brands and can combine their manufacturing across brands, sometimes using off the shelf base formulas that are adjusted.

> *Mass produced products use synthetic chemicals to imitate the actions of natural ingredients.*

Botanical ingredients are not identical batch to batch, for example a specific crop yield one year could offer a slightly different colour or consistency year on year.

On an industrial scale each batch needs to be the same every time, which is why synthetic ingredients are often favoured in large scale manufacturing.

Synthetic ingredients are a relatively new concept in skincare. In the past skincare was made from natural ingredients.

When did the beauty industry start?

The use of personal cosmetics in some form or another has been around since ancient times. Historians can trace our use of beauty products and cosmetics back to the ancient Egyptians, many thousands of years BC.

Early beauty routines relied upon natural ingredients and many products were used for more than one purpose.

Beauty treatments also relied on an area's natural resources for local sourcing of ingredients. The concept of multi-purpose products is coming back into the spotlight, as well as local sourcing of ingredients.

The modern beauty industry only appeared around the nineteenth century with the creation of beauty brands and mass marketing, which were the beginnings of the globalised beauty industry we see today.

What is a cosmetic?

The term cosmetic product applies to a much wider category of products than just make-up.

Personal cosmetics as a category has many different classes of product, including skincare.

However, around the world the definition of 'cosmetic product' broadly means any substance or mixture intended to be placed in contact with the external parts of the human body (skin, hair, nails, lips) or teeth with a view to cleaning, perfuming, changing their appearance, correcting odours, protecting them, or keeping them in good condition.

How many cosmetic products do you use a day?

Have you ever considered how many personal cosmetic products you use on your skin every day?

Every product you use has multiple chemicals (chemicals can be natural or synthetic). The compound effect of this over the course of a day, month or year is that we are applying hundreds of different ingredients to our skin a year.

More than ever, we are interested in understanding what ingredients are and where they came from.

Even if you are a low user of personal cosmetics, once you add up your products (from cleanser, shower gel, shampoo, conditioner, deodorant, make-up, body lotion, face cream) and count up how many different products you use each, you may be surprised at how many products and chemicals you are using on a daily basis.

The awareness of personal cosmetics chemicals is not about feeling uncomfortable or worried.

Understanding cosmetic ingredients is about having clarity and feeling empowered to know what you are putting on your skin. Get to know the ingredients in your products. Make informed decisions.

What things are listed on a skincare label?

Much of the information contained on our personal cosmetics is a legal requirement. Skincare labels are great sources of information and are often overlooked.

Some of the common information we will find include:

- Brand name
- Product name
- Product purpose and description
- Ingredient list (INCI)
- Product weight or volume
- Usage/storage directions
- Manufacturer's contact details.

Next time you are using a skincare product take a minute to look at the information on the label.

Why read skincare labels?

Many of us of are used to reading the ingredient list on the foods we consume.

However, reading the ingredient list on our personal cosmetics is still a new and growing habit.

The ingredients list is a way of knowing what we are putting on our skin.

Cut through the marketing and branding and get to know and understand your skincare product.

The only way to know what is in the products you are using is to read the ingredients label.

Many skincare products may contain ingredients that we are looking to avoid, such as ingredients that can be sensitising and irritating.

Sometimes we may want to support an independent brand or skincare manufactured in specific territory. British manufactured products are often appealing to specific territories overseas as a hallmark of trust.

Branding and packaging can make us think that a skincare product is something that it is not.

Many companies use a product name or label to highlight ingredients that are only present in tiny quantities.

In reality the quantities are not big enough for the ingredient to have an effect.

Also, terms such as 'natural' or 'organic' can be used by brands to give the impression that the product is made entirely from natural or organic ingredients when they are not.

> *To know what our skincare product is, we need to get into the habit of reading the ingredients list.*

Initially it can feel confusing however, as you get used to it, like with your food labels you will start to get more familiar with it. We also live in an age where we have access to almost instant information, so you are always able to research terms you want to know more about.

What is an INCI list?

The INCI list (pronounced "ink-ey") is the name given to the cosmetic ingredients list.

> *The INCI is the adopted way of stating ingredients on a skincare product.*

INCI is short for the International Nomenclature of Cosmetic Ingredients. It exists to help everyone easily identify ingredient in a product.

The INCI is often difficult to understand because natural ingredients are listed by their Latin names. This is a real challenge as it is hard to understand what that natural ingredient is, however, increasingly you will see the common name listed as well (because there is a growing demand by consumers wanting to understand what is going on their skin).

Synthetic ingredients do not use Latin names, they will just have their INCI name listed, however these scientific names can be quite tricky to work out given they are often long complex scientific words.

There are online resources and apps that can help you understand what these synthetic ingredients are, and some will even provide you additional safety information.

INCI ingredients are listed in order of their weight from the highest percentage to the lowest.

The ingredients that make up the bulk of your product are listed first. Ingredients which are included at 1% or lower are listed last but because they exist in such small amounts, there is no rule as to which order they are listed.

Are common allergens listed on the INCI?

Ingredients that commonly cause reactions for people with certain allergies or sensitivities, are listed last on the INCI. This is really helpful if you are sensitive to ingredients and want to quickly understand if there is an allergen in there that you want to avoid.

Allergens can be natural or synthetic, and they are found in many products.

Unless you have a specific issue, allergens are not always something you need to be worried about.

Even if these allergens are in tiny amounts, they must be listed there for people who know they have those allergies or those with particularly sensitive skin

The ingredients in a perfume or fragrance are often trade secrets, which means we do not know what ingredients are in them. However, if there is an allergen in them, it does have to be disclosed on the end of the INCI.

> *Taking an interest in the INCI is a good way of starting to understand what we are putting on our skin.*

It is also about being an empowered consumer.

What does 'clean' skincare mean?

The concept of clean skincare has been growing in recent years. However, it can be unclear what this term actually means.

> *Clean skincare is an unregulated term in the beauty industry*

Clean beauty is a term that is open to misuse by brands. It also carries with it the implication that some skincare products are clean while others are dirty or toxic, which isn't always helpful.

Clean skincare is ultimately about offering transparency about personal cosmetic ingredients

Transparency can be achieved in many ways. Some skincare brands achieve this with short ingredient lists, that are easy for consumers to understand others may set out a list of ingredients that they do not formulate with.

However, not every brand can agree on what ingredients are clean.

There is no one certifying body which tests and verifies that a product is clean, and it is left up to individual definition.

Understanding the cosmetic ingredients list is a key step in understanding what you are using.

Even though each company has a different definition of what clean skincare means, what is clear is that consumers are searching for products that will help them take control of their health and wellbeing.

It is also useful to know that in some territories cosmetic regulations are much looser than in others.

Clean beauty in one territory may have more consumer relevance in the context of the permitted inclusion of more harmful synthetic chemicals in personal cosmetics.

The US has quite different standards when it comes to personal cosmetics when compared to the EU and for this reason, the emergence of the clean beauty movement has strong roots in the US.

What is vegan skincare?

Vegan skincare still is a new and growing area in skincare. As consumer lifestyle habits change and more people embrace plant-based living, they are looking for alignment of their values across all the products they consume including their skincare.

Vegan skincare means that the product has no animal derived products in the formulation.

Historically there have been lots of animal by-products used in the formulation of cosmetics. Animal by-products such as lanolin, collagen, carmine, cholesterol, gelatine, honey, beeswax, and stearic acid can be found in many skincare products and cosmetics.

Moisturisers, soaps, and cleansers frequently include animal derived ingredients in their formulations.

Vegan skincare should also mean without animal testing, but this is not always the case in skincare products labelled as vegan.

Sometimes skincare products might be labelled as vegetarian friendly, which can lead us to believe that it does not contain animal products.

A vegetarian beauty or vegetarian skincare product does not have parts of an animal e.g., fat or gelatine from an animal. However, a vegetarian beauty product may still have animal by-products that are not part of the animal's body like lanolin or honey.

How can I tell if my skincare product is vegan?

To be sure that your skincare product is vegan look for brands and products that have vegan certification.

The Vegan Society accredited symbol means that products have been reviewed by an external party and the ingredients and production process have been scrutinised to ensure that they meet vegan standards.

Familiarising yourself with animal-derived ingredients and checking product ingredients lists is another way to find vegan-friendly products.

What is the difference between vegan and cruelty-free products?

Just because a skincare product is vegan does not necessarily mean it has not been tested on animals.

Not all cruelty-free skincare products are vegan.

A product that is cruelty free has not been tested on animals and does not contain ingredients tested on animals by another party.

The term 'cruelty-free' only refers to animal testing, it does not consider any ingredients that are derived from animals. So, for example a product might be cruelty free but contain carmine, a red pigment from crushed insects.

Cruelty free beauty products have not been tested on animals, do not have ingredients tested on animals but they may have animal derived ingredients.

What is minimalist skincare?

Mainstream skincare is often packed with lots of ingredients.

Synthetics, fragrance, cheap fillers, enhancers, and other potentially questionable ingredients.

It can often mean it is difficult to know if any are working or, more of a concern, what is irritating the skin.

Minimalist skincare is all about fewer ingredients and fewer products.

Minimalist skincare is about stripping skincare back to only what it really needs.

Using too many products in our skincare routine can run the risk of harming and weakening our skin barrier.

Paring back our routine to minimal products with fewer ingredients can help strengthen our skin while being gentle to the acid mantle, skin barrier and skin microbiome.

Simple is often better when it comes to skincare routines.

Not only is minimalist skincare kinder to our skin it can also be kinder to the environment. Minimalist skincare is generally low impact as it uses less resources from the planet.

What is waterless beauty?

Water scarcity is a major global crisis and the beauty industry like fast fashion is being forced to turn its attention to water.

Waterless beauty is a new area, and it means that the product does not have water in it as an ingredient.

Waterless formulations are often more concentrated than conventional beauty products. This is due to the lack of water in the formulation, which for some products can form the bulk of the ingredient list for a product.

Waterless beauty encompasses potent formulations, that have a beneficial impact on the skin.

If you have read the labels on our beauty products, you will have seen the word 'aqua' for water sitting right at the top for lots of products.

For many products water still makes up the bulk of the formulation. Even expensive serums can potentially have up to seventy per cent water.

You may also see beauty products labelled as waterless or formulations called 'water-free'.

These products are known as anhydrous (containing no water) formulations like balms and oils. You will not see 'Aqua' listed on the INCI.

However, even if a beauty product does not contain water all products do have a water footprint.

Products will have gone through the stages in the manufacturing, processing, or shipping that involve water.

Consumers of skincare products also have a water footprint from using products

The use of water is coming under scrutiny and this is an area that is set to develop further as we become more aware of waterless beauty and our water footprint.

What is organic skincare?

Organic skin care is generally defined as skin care products which contain organically grown ingredients that are grown without the use of Genetically Modified Organisms (GM), herbicides and synthetic fertilisers.

The difference between natural skin care and organic skin care?

Natural skincare products are those which contain ingredients that come from natural sources but are not necessarily organically produced.

They may be plant-based but those ingredients may not necessarily be grown according to organic practices.

Organic skincare also includes products from naturally sourced ingredients, but these are grown without synthetic chemicals or pesticides.

What is the meaning of certified organic?

Certified organic skincare products are those that have been certified by a third-party regulatory body, who set a certain number of production rules for organic certification.

The certifying body may vary territory to territory.

Are cosmetics tested on animals?

The use of animals to test cosmetics products or their ingredients is banned in the UK and the European Union.

Cosmetic products sold in Europe are not tested on animals.

However, this is not the case for all countries around the world.

Although several countries outside the UK and EU are also now looking to adopt similar bans, others including China and the United States of America, still use animals to test cosmetics ingredients and products.

What is cruelty free beauty?

A product that is labelled cruelty-free is one that has been produced without any form of animal testing throughout the creation and production process.

To be sure look for third party cruelty free certification.

What is sustainable skincare?

Green issues in the beauty industry are becoming mainstream and sustainability is at the forefront of many consumers.

Sustainable skincare satisfies the needs of the present without compromising the future.

There are three broad pillars of sustainability: environment, social and economic.

Here are ways in which a beauty brand may be embracing sustainability:

- Sustainable packaging
- Organic/sustainable ingredients
- Ethical /sustainable sourcing and production
- Waste management
- Supporting Fairtrade
- Supporting local economies

Sustainable skincare will often use environmentally friendly formulations, production practices or packaging methods.

Are skincare products biodegradable?

The future of skin care is starting to focus more on sustainability and consumers are increasingly looking for biodegradable products to help reduce their overall impact on the planet.

The term biodegradation explains the naturally occurring breakdown of materials by microorganisms.

Whilst there is no fixed timeline for it, essentially if something is biodegradable it can be broken down over time through the action of naturally occurring microorganisms (such as bacteria, fungi, and algae).

Composting is a similar but different process that is much more familiar to the average consumer.

Consumers are interested in understanding whether their skin care products are biodegradable.

The biodegradability of a skincare formulation is a different thing to whether the packaging is biodegradable. Many of our skin care products will end up being washed off our skin and go down the drain to be processed as wastewater.

Not all ingredients used in personal care are biodegradable.

Synthetic ingredients, silicones and synthetics additives and fragrances are not easily biodegradable and can affect aquatic environments.

What are microplastics?

Plastic particles found within many personal care products will take hundreds, or even thousands of years to break down into harmless molecules. During that time, the consequences for the surrounding environment can be dire.

From textiles (called microfibres) and exfoliating scrubs (called microbeads) to silicones and petrochemicals, plastics are everywhere when it comes to personal care and cosmetic products.

Microplastics are so tiny, most people are not even aware that the products they are using contain these microplastic and that every time they wash their face little particles are rinsing away down the drain and into the wastewater systems, which can then find their way into streams, rivers, and the world's oceans.

Sometimes the sludge that accumulates from these nondegradable ingredients is even used as fertiliser for crops.

What is green chemistry in skincare?

Green chemistry is about incorporating sustainable principles into the practices of creating and manufacturing skincare products.

Green chemistry is a set of twelve principles that are aimed at helping the cosmetics and personal care industry to strive toward greener processes and products.

What is green washing?

Green washing is when a product or company makes claims to be natural, eco-friendly, organic, or environmentally conscious when they are not any of those things.

Greenwashing can be done through marketing, advertising, product descriptions, company name or the use of images or packaging design that would make consumers believe the product is green, natural, or sustainable.

By being an educated consumer and doing your research you can avoid being green washed.

Seek out companies and retailers that publish their standards and benchmarks and who make information accessible.

There are more legitimate green beauty products and brands out there than ever before, so take the time to support the genuine ones.

What are non-comedogenic products?

Non-comedogenic is the umbrella term used to describe products that do not have pore-clogging ingredients

Pores play a vital role in releasing sweat and toxins from the body and if they are blocked, the skin can become congested and irritated.

Pores also regulate our skin's production of sebum oil. The right amount of sebum keeps skin soft and supple, too much can leave the skin oily and attract acne related bacteria.

> *Not all brands state that they are non-comedogenic on their product labels.*

If you are unsure whether a product is non-comedogenic, look for clues on the product's INCI list (ingredients label).

Bulky petrochemical mineral oils and shiny silicones are pore-clogging, and they are commonly added to skin care products. Once applied to the skin they act like a layer of cling-film, trapping dirt in and hindering the skin from breathing, naturally.

What happens if cosmetics are not preserved?

All products containing water need to be preserved.

Products that are naturally hostile to microorganisms such as those without water, with a low or high pH, or with a high alcohol content are however, unlikely to have microorganisms growing them.

For all other products, preservatives are included in cosmetic products to ensure the shelf life of the products and to protect the product from any external factors that might compromise the safety of the product.

How do companies test their skincare products?

Once a skincare product has been formulated, challenge testing is a common method used to test the effectiveness of the preservative against the certain types of pathogenic microorganisms in cosmetics.

Challenge testing involves deliberately contaminating the formulated skincare product with specific microorganisms and observing their growth.

Before a new skin care product can be launched, the formulation is tested in several separate ways.

The formulation must be challenged and checked to ensure that the consumer who uses it will not come to any harm.

The testing phase is often complex and time-consuming and involves checking many different physical and chemical properties of the formulation.

> ## Checks may also be carried out to ensure that claims made about the product are substantiated.

In addition, the safety of every chemical ingredient in the formulation must be checked by suitably qualified experts to ensure that they will not cause any harm to the consumer using the product.

This phase in the development and launch of a new product is usually known as the safety or risk assessment phase.

It may seem that the launch of a skincare product is the end of the testing process, but brand owners always keep each product that they sell under watch.

This process is often known as post market surveillance and it's designed so that brand owners can spot the products that may be causing problems for those who are using them.

What is stability testing?

During the development of a skincare product the cosmetic scientist will identify a number of microbiological and chemical attributes that will be used to set the quality standards for the product.

Uniform global testing methods will then be used to measure each of these characteristics against specific standards.

These testing methods and standards are referred to as stability testing.

Compliance with the standards ensures that the consumer can use the product in the knowledge that they will not cause them any harm during the time that the product is being used.

This is a principle that underpins stability testing of a new cosmetic product.

What is microbiological testing?

Skincare products are made in different ways and then used and stored by consumers.

As a result, they can be at risk of becoming contaminated by microorganisms such as bacteria and moulds.

Strict criteria have been developed by both cosmetic companies and government regulators to prevent cosmetic products becoming affected by microorganisms.

Before launching a product for use by consumers, the microbiological quality of the ingredients and the end product must be satisfactory.

What is a safety assessment?

Your skincare products will undergo a safety assessment before you can buy them.

It is a fundamental requirement that cosmetic products are safe.

Skincare products must not cause any harm to consumers whatever their age gender or ethnic origin.

In many countries of the world brand owners are obliged by local laws to ensure the safety of ingredients and their finished products.

Formulations go through a structured review process, that involves a detailed check of the products and ingredients by a qualified expert cosmetic safety assessor.

The process is often known as a risk or safety assessment.

The EU has been at the forefront in developing this philosophy as applied to cosmetic products.

The first step of the risk or safety assessment process is to have the details of the ingredients checked by a qualified expert safety assessor to confirm whether the ingredients are likely to cause any harm to consumers.

4 Decode Your Skincare

What products you choose to buy is down to personal choice and needs.

However, more people are looking into natural skincare and questioning the need for synthetic ingredients, and this is for lots of different reason.

Sometimes people are looking to avoid potentially irritating synthetic chemicals.

Others feel unsure about the long-term safety of some of the ingredients in products they use.

Some simply want to seek out brands and natural products that match their values.

Natural ingredients can be a way to connect with nature or return to something a little bit simpler.

What is natural skin care?

The term natural in skincare does not have a set definition within the industry, which causes a lot of problems as natural can means different things.

For most people natural skincare implies that the products are formulated with ingredients found in nature, such as from plants, seeds and nuts and are without any synthetic ingredients.

> *The best way to ensure a product is natural is to look at the ingredients list.*

As a consumer a lot depends on your personal choice and interest in learning about ingredients.

When considering if something is natural you can look at what the ingredient is derived from (is it from a natural source) and how has it been processed.

Naturally occurring ingredients are ones that are presented in their natural, unprocessed state.

Naturally derived, physically processed ingredients (naturally occurring ingredients which have been processed using physical processes such as cold-pressing or filtration). For example, cold-pressed oils, distillation of flowers to produce essential oils.

Naturally derived, chemically processed ingredients are naturally occurring ingredients which have been synthetically processed to become an entirely different chemical and structural substance.

What is meant by synthetic ingredients in skincare?

Synthetic skincare means products that incorporate laboratory and scientifically derived ingredients.

Synthetic skincare formulas are made using chemical copies of natural ingredients. These are ingredients which have been created and processed in a lab.

Why choose natural skincare?

An increasing number of people are interested in the ingredients that they are putting on their skin and many are choosing natural extracts from plants over synthetic chemicals.

By choosing natural skincare products over synthetics, many feel more comfortable with the chemical compounds that they are applying to their skin on a daily basis.

Natural products can be particularly beneficial for people who suffer from skin sensitivities.

Skin irritations and sensitivities are often triggered by artificial fragrances, alcohol, parabens, and synthetic foaming agents, all of which are common in traditional skincare products.

Making the switch to a natural skincare routine can help cut a lot of common irritants from your routine, reducing the risk of flare ups, and working to naturally heal and soothe skin sensitivities.

From an ecological perspective natural skincare can have a better impact on the environment once it has been used. Our personal cosmetics end up in the waterways after use. They are washed off and this goes down your sink, shower or drain.

The by-products of your personal cosmetics end up back in the eco-system.

Natural skin care products are bio-compatible and can return to nature with no long-term harm.

Synthetic chemicals do not all disappear when they enter the ecosystem, and they can cause complications and impact the marine biosphere.

Regulation of synthetic skincare can vary territory to territory so natural skincare can offer more transparency and control over what you are putting on your skin.

There is a growing debate that continues around the impact of synthetic compounds in skincare to impact the balance of our hormones.

Synthetic skincare products are able to easily add cheap chemicals diluted in filler ingredients to bulk up the mix to increase profits.

With natural skincare products it is harder to bulk out the formulation and every single part is included for a reason.

Since those ingredients are more potent, it takes less product to have efficacy.

Synthetic skin care products can cause rashes, inflammation, irritation and itch, and other symptoms of allergies.

> *People are growing increasingly mindful about what they put on their skin.*

Some people believe that synthetic chemicals are better for the skin than natural ingredients, because of the misconception that powerful active skincare needs to have synthetic chemicals to be effective.

However, natural products and ingredients can be as potent if not more so than their synthetic counterpart.

With so many effective, accessible natural skin care solutions readily available, now is the time to consider a natural approach to skincare.

Do cosmetic products get absorbed beyond the skin?

Cosmetic products do most of their work on the surface of the skin.

Moisturisation, one of the main functions of skincare has the most effect in maintaining the healthy appearance of the topmost layer of skin.

However, many people are concerned about if and how deep skincare products and their ingredients penetrate the skin.

The skin acts primarily as a barrier to prevent foreign material from entering. There is evidence that certain molecules do have the ability to travel through the stratum corneum and epidermis. For example, transdermal drug patches such as nicotine can reach the bloodstream.

> ## *It is important to know that it is difficult for ingredients to penetrate beyond the stratum corneum.*

The skin is an exceptionally good barrier in most instances that does not let materials into the cell.

To reach lower levels of the skin any ingredient must travel through a complicated long journey before it can potentially influence structural components. However, this journey is difficult, and most skincare ingredients stay on or in the stratum corneum.

Some small molecules (such as peptides and retinoids) can penetrate deeper into the skin, where they have the potential to bring about cosmetic change.

It is important to know that cosmetic products must not have a long-term physiological function on the skin, or it then becomes a drug not a cosmetic.

There are a lot of different associated regulations around drug development, which make this a quite different discipline and cosmetic products must not cross this line.

What is the difference between mineral oils and plant oils?

Plant based facial oils are great for skin and they can be extracted from a range of different plants, seeds, and nuts.

Plant oils have a rich range of colours, aromas, and properties.

Plant oils are gentle on our skin and can help our microbiome to flourish through working effectively with our skin's flora.

Plant oils can help reduce the amount of water that evaporates off the skin to minimise trans-epidermal water loss, however they are often more expensive and precious when compared to mineral oil.

Mineral oil is a cheap ingredient and it is found in many personal cosmetic products. It is a highly refined and purified and belongs to a class of chemicals called hydrocarbons (which includes petrolatum, paraffin, and mineral oil). Mineral oil is widely used as emollients in products, because of their low volatility and smoothing texture.

Mineral oil is widespread in skincare and despite its low cost it can be found as a filler in many expensive prestige products too.

> *Mineral oil is derived from petroleum, it does not absorb into the skin, as its molecular size is excessively big.*

Mineral oil when used in skincare stays on the surface of the skin. It can clog the pores and it not like plant oils that can penetrate the skin to fortify the skin barrier.

Plant based oils supply nutrients vitamins, essential fatty acids, and antioxidants to protect and fortify the lipid barrier in our skin. Mineral oils on the other hand have none of these benefits.

Why is palm oil used in skincare?

Palm oil is a form of vegetable oil from the fruit of the oil palm tree. It has recently become one of the world's most widely produced oils and is a key ingredient in many cosmetic products.

However, to make room for palm tree plantations, tropical rainforests have been cleared on a massive scale and deforestation and the loss of natural habitats has a devastating impact on the planet.

Palm oil is in a lot of personal cosmetics, in part because it is cheap and a uniquely effective vegetable fat.

HEALTHY SKIN x HEALTHY VIBES

Palm oil is used within thousands of ingredients and has become deeply entrenched in the personal care industry.

A lot of consumers now wish to avoid using products containing palm oil but there is extraordinarily little transparency to the consumer. Often, we are unaware that palm oil is used in a product we are using.

Once an ingredient such as palm oil has been altered synthetically through a chemical process, it can be called by its new chemical name. The industry relies heavily on these synthetic ingredients as emulsifiers, thickeners, surfactants (cleansers), and preservatives.

Many products that use palm oil are not clearly labelled as such.

Palm oil and its derivatives can appear under many names, including:

Vegetable Oil, Vegetable Fat, Palm Kernel, Palm Kernel Oil, Palm Fruit Oil, Palmate, Palmitate, Palmolein, Glyceryl, Stearate, Stearic Acid, Elaeis Guineensis, Palmitic Acid, Palm Stearine, Palmitoyl Oxostearamide, Palmitoyl Tetrapeptide-3, Sodium Laureth Sulfate, Sodium Lauryl Sulfate, Sodium Kernelate, Sodium Palm Kernelate, Sodium Lauryl Lactylate/Sulphate, Hyrated Palm Glycerides, Etyl Palmitate, Octyl Palmitate, Palmityl Alcohol.

If you wish to avoid palm oil all together look for brands that are clear in their messaging that they are palm-oil free.

What is oxidative stress?

Oxidative stress is natural process that happens in our bodies as a by-product of cell reactions or under a number of conditions such as exposure to UV, cigarette smoke and air pollution.

When oxidative stress occurs, we end up with free radicals roaming around in our cells. These are unstable molecules looking for an electron.

Stable molecules have pairs of electrons in their outer rings, but free radicals are one electron short and they fix this by stealing an electron from the next closest molecule to complete itself.

When this happens a chain reaction is started, which if not stopped can damage skin cells, collagen, and even strains of DNA.

Antioxidants are helpful as they are molecules with an electron to spare, sharing it with the free radical before it can cause any damage, and remaining stable itself.

Lots of foods include antioxidants, which is where we primarily derive them from.

However, when looking at improving skin conditions it's worth bringing them into our skincare routines as well.

Our body purposely creates free radicals to neutralise viruses and bacteria. However, too much of it can affect the DNA, lipids and proteins that can trigger diseases.

These free radicals are unstable, highly reactive molecules that have unpaired electrons.

To gain stability, they attack stable molecules, triggering a chain reaction that damages healthy cells.

Once an overload of free radicals is present in our system, it causes oxidative stress, or an imbalance between the production of free radicals and the ability of the body to counteract or detoxify their harmful effects.

Environmental factors like radiation from the sun, pollution, radiation, cigarette smoke and other toxic chemicals are also known to trigger the formation of free radicals.

What are AHAs?

Alpha Hydroxy Acids also known as AHAs offer chemical exfoliation as an alternative to manual exfoliation.

AHAs work by helping to dissolve the bonds between skin cells to allow the removal of dead cells and revealing a smoother skin surface.

AHAs are a class of chemical compounds that can be either naturally occurring or synthetic.

Low concentrations are suitable for home use, but chemical peels contain much higher concentrations so must be used under the supervision of a professional.

What are enzymes?

Enzymes help dissolve and unglue the bonds between dead skin cells, which causes skin to exfoliate and slough off.

Enzymes in skincare are usually derived from plant sources and they are found in exfoliating products.

> *Enzymes help exfoliate without disrupting our pH which means they are great for skin health*

Enzymes are the gentlest form of exfoliation, making them ideal for sensitive complexions.

Are AHAs and enzymes the only chemical exfoliants?

There are a range of acids that can be used in chemical exfoliates, BHAs and PHAs (both types of acid) are also popular acids in skincare.

BHAs (beta-hydroxy acids) like salicylic acid, 'unglue' the bonds holding dull, dead skin on the surface, and PHAs (polyhydroxy acids) are similar to AHAs, but potentially less sensitising on the skin.

Who are AHAs best suited to?

AHAs tend to provide quick results, but also have the potential to irritate the skin.

They are best used with caution if you have sensitive skin if the product has a high percentage of acid.

Are enzymes better than acids?

If you like your skincare to be gentle, then enzymes are potentially preferable to certain types of acids.

Enzymes are a much gentler way to exfoliate and brighten the complexion, and especially beneficial for those with sensitive skin.

In general, acids like AHAs and BHAs are more potent and work more deeply and intensely and with that come more potential for irritation.

> *Enzymes are a great choice for those who find they are unable to tolerate acids and need a gentler touch.*

Pomegranate, papaya, and pumpkin are at the forefront of enzymatic exfoliation.

Pomegranate is also hailed for its brightening properties, so using products with papaya enzymes will help diminish age spots and even help brighten up our complexion.

Who are enzymes best suited to?

Enzymes are by far the gentlest form of exfoliation and suitable for those who suffers with some sensitivity.

Enzymes work slower than AHAs and can be incorporated into our everyday skin regime with no damage to our skin barrier health.

What animal ingredients are in skincare?

As more people become aware of vegan skincare, many people are coming to realise that personal cosmetics may contain ingredients from animals or animal by-products.

Here are some examples of how animals and animal by-products are used in personal cosmetics:

Tallow
Rendered animal fat that comes from boiling an animal's carcass. It can be found as a base to many cosmetics.

Hyaluronic Acid
When animal-derived, a protein found in umbilical cords and the fluids around the joints of animals.

Keratin
Protein from the ground-up horns, hooves, feathers, quills, and hair of various animals.

Gelatine
A thickening agent derived from boiled skin, tendons, ligaments, and bones of animals and used in creamy products.

Collagen
A protein from animal tissue. Is often used in skincare for plumping effect.

Retinol
Does not always have to be from an animal derived source, but often is. Is a fat-soluble derivative of vitamin A found mostly in animal foods like oily fish and liver.

Stearic Acid
When animal-derived, a fat from cows, pigs, and sheep.

Carmine
A red pigment collected from crushed insects. Found in blushers, lipsticks, and cosmetics.

Lanolin
An animal wax produced by woolly animals like sheep.

Ambergris
Produced in the digestive system of sperm whales, it's commonly used in perfume.

How do adaptogens benefit skin?

Adaptogens, a group of naturally medicinal herbs and botanicals that have their roots in traditional Ayurvedic and Chinese medicine.

Adaptogens are specific herbs and botanicals that offer medicinal support to the body in managing and adapting to the internal effects of stress on our system.

Adaptogens can help skin as part of a comprehensive approach to stress management.

Our skin does not do well under extended periods of imbalance or stress in the body, which can result in a reduced barrier function, hormone-related breakouts, elasticity loss and oxidative stress.

By helping to normalise how certain systems in the body respond to stress (such the adrenal glands which regulate hormones) adaptogens may help get things back to better health.

If you are looking for adaptogens in your skincare notable herbs include Indian gooseberry/Amla fruit and ashwagandha.

What are parabens used for?

Parabens are a family of preservatives and you will find them on cosmetic labels listed as methyl-, ethyl-, propyl- and butylparaben, or in their salt form, listed as methylparaben.

Parabens are added to formulations containing water to kill or inhibit the growth of pathogens. They are used to give items a longer shelf life and stop bacteria from growing within products.

Should you avoid parabens?

There has been a lot of concern in recent years around whether parabens pose a risk to our health or not.

Parabens are believed to disrupt hormone function by mimicking oestrogen. Too much oestrogen can trigger an increase in breast cell division and growth of tumours, which is why paraben use has been linked to breast cancer and reproductive issues. There is a lot that has been written about whether these studies on parabens are sufficiently credible, however the debate over parabens continues.

In most territories' parabens are not a banned ingredient.

It is important you make up your own mind about parabens. For some people, parabens are an ingredient they want to actively avoid, and many skincare products do not use parabens in their formulations.

How can you avoid parabens?

To really understand what is in your skin care product you need to read the ingredient lists.

If you are looking to avoid parabens in your skincare the kinds of ingredients you will be looking for is methylparaben, butylparaben, propylparaben or isoparaben. This will show that a product has parabens.

Should you avoid fragrance in your skincare?

Fragrances are complex mixtures of natural and synthetic chemicals that come together to make a particular smell in our products.

They can be made from all synthetic materials in a lab or all plant derived oils and extracts, or a mixture of both.

You may see fragrance listed as "fragrance" or "parfum" on ingredient labels.

———————

Fragrance is usually toward the bottom of an ingredient list as it is only needed in small quantities to be effective.

While most ingredients need to be listed out one by one, fragrance mixtures can simply be labelled as "fragrance" in products because they are trade secrets in the cosmetics industry.

This makes "fragrance" difficult for us to decipher what ingredients in that fragrance might be triggering allergies or sensitivities.

Fragrance has come under fire because we don't always have full visibility of the ingredients that go into them.

———————

As a result, increasingly more people are turning to "fragrance-free" skincare to avoid skin irritations and fragrance sensitivity.

What is CBD skincare?

CBD (also known as cannabidiol) is the non-intoxicating component of marijuana or hemp plants.

CBD is extracted as a powder, and is typically mixed with an oil like olive, hemp, or coconut, all of which enhance application and effectiveness.

CBD oil in skincare will not get you high because it does not have the mind-altering properties of marijuana's tetrahydrocannabinol (THC) content.

It's extracted from the leaves of the hemp plant whose THC content is exceptionally low. CBD in skincare is used to soothe and calm the skin

What is the difference between hemp and CBD?

Hemp seed oil is an omega-rich oil sourced from the seeds of the hemp plant (also known as the cannabis sativa plant). These seeds do not contain calming cannabinoid and generally only contain trace amounts of CBD.

Cannabidiol (CBD) is sourced from cannabis leaves. It's rich in cannabinoids and contains minimal THC.

CBD helps restore overall balance in the body along with other benefits. CBD can be sourced from both marijuana and hemp plants.

5 Skin & Wellness

Skin care is a form of self-care and it forms part of our wellness and wellbeing, which are about how we live our life. Skin care however, is not a substitute for medical attention.

A skincare routine may help us to improve the appearance of our skin, however there is also a self-care aspect to this daily routine.

When you take ten minutes out of your day in the morning and evening to look after your skin, you are doing soothing and comforting things for yourself and that is a type of self-care.

The process of caring for your skin can be relaxing and calming if you allow it to be.

Self-care can mean different things to each individual, but the goal of any act of selfcare is to feel good, happy, and calm and to improve how we feel overall.

You do not need to be a skin care junkie to embrace self-care through your daily routine. The important thing is to take time for yourself and our skin reflects our over-all wellness.

What is holistic skin care?

Holistic skin care is taking a lifestyle and comprehensive approach to health and balance.

A holistic health approach to skincare means looking at and treating skin health as a whole, and not just parts of it. It means looking for the causes as opposed to simply just treating symptoms.

Holistic skin care acknowledges that our environment and inner imbalances (physical, emotional, mental) can have profound consequences for our health including our skin and we need to take everything into account if we would like to restore that balance.

We should aspire to improve our overall wellbeing.

Prevention, positive lifestyle changes, determining underlying causes of a bad condition, and treating the body as a system of interrelated parts are just as critical to supporting health as skincare or treatments.

In the case of skin care, a holistic approach means putting on a product on our face is not enough.

It only treats one part of the skin and the overall health of our skin depends on more than that.

It's not enough to treat it from the outside only. We have to nurture it from the inside as well.

How our skin looks and feels depends on many factors. From the ingredients we use in our cosmetics, through to our lifestyle choices such as diet and exercise, the environmental stressors we meet, to our emotional and mental wellbeing.

How to think of your skin care holistically?

Here are some tips for how to think of your skin through a holistic lens.

- Get familiar with your own skin. Look, feel, and observe your skin though out the months, over seasons and how it performs in different situations.

- Know what your skin is like and what it needs to choose the best ingredients and products.

- Learn how to decode an ingredient list.

- Skin care is a long-term game and is meant to nurture the skin inside and out.

- Cosmetic products cannot fix underlying causes of acne.

- Nothing will magically reverse the ageing process.

- Stay away from harsh, stripping products.

- Try a good oil-based cleanser to preserve the vital barrier function of the skin.

- Use good vitamins and antioxidants that are proven to work.

- Wear SPF.

- And most importantly, establish a skin care routine.

Give your skin the care it deserves every single day.

How does stress effect our skin?

Stress is bad for us and it shows on our skin.

It can lead to acne flare-ups, hives, rashes, hair loss or can increase and worsen existing skin conditions.

Stress can cause us to break out it causes our body to make hormones like cortisol, which tells glands in our skin to make more oil.

It can also be stressful to have problems with our skin. We may feel anxious or upset about how our skin is looking and feeling, which adds more stress.

There are all kinds of stresses, physical, emotional, psychological, and environmental and our skin is influenced by each of them.

Cortisol

Feeling stressed causes an upsurge in our levels of cortisol which can then raise sugar levels in the blood and sebum levels. It activates sebaceous glands in the skin, leading to blocked pores and acne breakouts.

Everything becomes oilier. It also makes our skin more reactive and sensitive, and healing can take longer.

Adrenaline

When we are stressed, we experience a spike in adrenaline, which causes us to sweat more. Skin can become quickly dehydrated which leads to loss of tone, fullness, and smoothness.

Cortisol and adrenaline can give skin a combination of problems. It becomes dry and flaky in some places and congested and oily in others.

Stress can also:

- Cause flare-ups of existing problems like rosacea, eczema, and psoriasis.
- Disrupt the balance of good and bad bacteria in our gut which then also causes breakouts.
- Affect our quality of sleep, which affects our skin.
- Trigger inflammation because our body feels under attack and inflammatory cells increase in number, and flare-ups begin.

What can we do to help manage stress?

- Improving the quality of our sleep is important when managing stress.

- Make space for mindful relaxation, get some exercise and fresh air, and eat as healthily as we can.

- To help our skin, adopt a skincare routine with a small number of products that work gently together, and which will not overwhelm your skin.

- Stressed skin needs to be cleansed properly to remove excess sebum without drying it out.

- Stressed skin needs to be soothed.

How does sleep improve our skin?

When we sleep our skin has time for the skin cells to regenerate.

In the day, our skin is fighting UV rays, pollution, sweat and grime.

While we are sleeping, our skin moves into recovery mode and we should think of it as valuable time of repair and regeneration.

The skin regeneration process at night is much faster than during the day.

When we sleep our skin can be more receptive to products.

Once we fall asleep, our body produces growth hormones which also help your skin in producing enough collagen, which helps your skin remain tight and bouncy.

When we sleep it also allows our skin to repair acne and scarring.

Sleep is a great stress-reliever for your mind and body and your skin too.

What are the skin benefits of drinking water?

Drinking water helps the whole body, from flushing out toxins to preventing acne and giving us glowing skin.

When we drink enough water, the cells in our body get hydrated and the skin also gets hydrated.

Here are all the benefits of drinking water for our skin:

Improves Skin Tone

Drinking enough water helps the body to flush out toxins while giving us healthier skin.

Prevents Premature Ageing

Staying hydrated helps increase elasticity in the skin as it stays moisturised for longer. Heightened elasticity in the skin delays sagging of the skin and no premature appearance of fine lines and wrinkles.

Reduces Puffiness

When the skin looks puffy, it can be retaining water to protect us from dehydration. This occurs when we don't drink enough water. Staying hydrated will reduce swelling and puffiness in our face.

Prevents Acne

Drinking water help balance the oil and water content on the skin of our face. This helps to prevent excess oil and sebum secretion, which means fewer clogged pores and acne.

What are the benefits of a good diet on our skin?

How we eat is just as important when it comes to skin care as what we put onto our skin. We cannot expect to have healthy skin if our diet is poor and inadequate.

> *The healthier and more balanced our diet is, the more it will show in our skin.*

Skin care products can help nurture the skin, but without a healthy diet these effects will be limited and will not last for an extended period.

The things we eat has a much greater impact on the overall appearance and condition of our skin.

A healthy diet includes raw minerals, vitamins, other nutrients, acids, phytochemicals, and other useful compounds that our skin and body need daily.

Moisturising effects

Skin dryness is one of the most common skin and poor diet can lead to this issue. A healthy diet means eating enough healthy fats.

Essential fatty acids help preserve the moisture and suppleness of our skin.

They keep the skin moisturised naturally both inside and out. Avocados, seeds, nuts, and olive oil are examples of healthy fats.

Prevent wrinkles

A healthy diet can help optimise the production of collagen (crucial for the elasticity of the skin) and the health of skin cells. One of the ways in which a proper diet can stabilise the production of collagen in the body is by cutting down the amount of sugar and white carbs that we eat.

Help with acne

A healthy diet can help people prevent and eliminate acne particularly of we reduce our consumption of sugar. Consume more healthy fats, lean protein, and leafy green veggies and avoid sugar to fight acne.

Makes our skin brighter

When we don't take care of what we eat and drink, our skin can look lifeless and dull. This is because an improper diet means that there are some crucial nutrients and compounds missing. We should aim to consume healthy, natural fruits and vegetables foods and replace processed foods with natural unprocessed foods.

How does our gut health impact our skin?

Our gut is filled with bacteria (like our skin microbiome) that influences our body's digestive response and our immune system function.

The gut microbiome is made up of trillions of bacteria and microorganisms. We still have a lot to learn about the connection between our gut and our skin however research is showing that there is a connection between our gut health and our skin, called the gut-skin axis.

Our diet and the impact of that on our gut health has a direct impact on the health of our skin.

If we want to have healthy skin, then we should be looking after our gut microbiota to help our skin flourish.

If you want to build a healthy gut microbiome that can help maintain healthy skin, you may want to consider adding more probiotics and prebiotics to your diet (which help stimulate growth of certain healthy bacteria in the gut).

The gut-skin axis is not a new concept (even though modern research may make us think it is). Traditional forms of medicine that have been around for thousands of years, such as Ayurvedic medicine and traditional Chinese medicine, have always placed focus on internal health.

How can exercise help skin health?

Exercise can help ease stress and release feel-good hormones, like endorphins that regulate the stress hormone cortisol (also responsible for acne-causing oil production and inflammation).

Sweating during exercise can also help clear out the skin.

Exercise also helps improves circulation and blood flow, which is vital for carrying away waste products and transporting oxygen and nutrients to skin cells.

Moving our bodies also promotes better sleep, which brings us back to better skin.

How is skin care self-care?

Skin care routines can play an important health aspect to our overall wellbeing. Skincare is self-care.

The benefits of a daily skin care routine go beyond appearances.

It does not matter if that is taking a few minutes to yourself to use a face mask, quietly cleansing your face or massaging in a facial oil at bedtime.

Having a set routine every day, you know what to expect and for some people this routine provides a lot of relief.

The more a of a routine your skin care becomes, the less stress it is.

―――――――

Not everyone begins a skin care routine for beauty reasons. The act of looking out for our skin, can be comforting and soothing.

We are often alone when doing our skin care routine, in our bedroom, bathroom or somewhere quiet.

Taking 10 minutes out of your day for you can be calming.

A skin care routine also gives you a chance to take a break from whatever the day is throwing at you and put everything on pause.

There is no limit to what skincare routines or rituals are considered self-care.

Why are facial workouts good?

At-home facial workouts are starting to become popular as they are easy to do and can result in lots of healthy skin benefits. Just like going to the gym these are workouts for the muscles in your face.

A facial workout aims to use movement to tone your muscles, reduce fine lines, increase blood circulation, and release tension.

As with all workouts if we want results the trick is consistency.

Your face contains over fifty different muscles and a lot of facial muscles are rarely used.

Carrying out regular facial exercises, helps promote the circulation of blood to the different areas of the face and replenishing the oxygen supply in the muscles and the skin.

This affects complexion and can help us develop a naturally healthy glow.

Gua sha is a face massage tool that is considered a natural therapy and it has been used in traditional Chinese medicine as far back as the Ming Dynasty. It involves using a gua sha tool to scrap your skin to improve your circulation.

A gua sha tool is often made of out of rose quartz, jade, as well as other materials and it is a small, contoured tool designed to fit the contours of our face.

The gua sha massage tool can be used after applying a facial oil to stimulate deeper absorption and hydration. The facial oil helps the tool to also glide more easily over our face.

Facial massage promotes lymphatic drainage, relaxes tension and regular use can help smooth, tone and brighten our skin

Massage helps improve to blood flow and stimulate collagen production.

Using a gua sha tool allows us to work on our skin with a light or firm pressure, depending on how we are feeling.

We can also keep our gua sha in the fridge for a cooling massage to reduce puffiness.

What is the benefit of using a gua sha tool?

- Relaxing muscles
- Getting energy and blood moving
- Reducing puffiness
- Encouraging healthy circulation
- Eliminating toxins
- Encouraging the skin to make new collagen

How to use a gua sha tool for face massage?

Smooth a few drops of plant facial oil onto your face and neck and lightly massage it in.

Starting on the neck, place the gua sha on your neck and pull down gently using an even, sweeping stroke in a downwards motion from under our ear to the top of our collar bone.

Work your way along the front of our neck and through to the other side and repeat two or three times.

From the centre of your chin pull out towards your ear along the jawline and gently support the skin with your other hand on your chin.

> *For a deeper massage use the V-shape of the gua sha tool to work along the jawline.*

Moving on to your cheeks, press down from the side of our nose towards your ear. Repeat this a few times on each side.

Using the tip of the gua sha, place it underneath your eye and using sweeping motions, gently move outwards towards the temple. This area is delicate so be gentle.

Finish by working from the centre of the brows and move upwards towards the hairline, slowly working out from here and repeating two or three times.

Why try facial massage?

Facial massages are treatments we can do on our own. The technique involves stimulating pressure points on the face, neck, and shoulders.

> *We can use oil, or cleansing balms with facial massages, as well as a face roller or a gua sha tool.*

Facial massage helps promote healthy skin while relaxing our facial muscles.

It has a relaxing and rejuvenating effect, helping us look and feel better.

Whether we want to use facial massage purely for relaxation or to treat a specific condition, there are plenty of techniques to explore and try at home.

What is face yoga?

Face yoga is about exercising your face rather than your body. It involves a facial exercise routine where you make repetitive motions and exaggerated facial expressions to strengthen different muscle groups in your face. The aim of this is to keep the skin on top of our faces looking and feeling plump and firm.

Our faces have over fifty muscles and some of these are rarely used.

Face yoga looks to tone and work more muscles in your face to help lift and tighten the skin over time. When practised regularly, face yoga can help to build a holistic sense of wellbeing and mindfulness similar to yoga or meditation.

How to practice slow beauty?

Slow beauty is part of a lifestyle which prioritises health, physical and mental wellbeing, the environment, and the wider community.

It is part of a cultural shift of living life and doing things more slowly and more mindfully.

Slow beauty is an extension of the slow living movement, which was a backlash to over consumption and fast living. You may have heard of slow food and slow fashion; slow beauty is part of that way of thinking.

It is not just a lifestyle choice, slow beauty is a necessity. Global warming is becoming an increasing threat, the awareness of the need to protect the environment is continuing to grow and slow beauty is part of the narrative that surrounds consumption and what impact that has on people and the planet.

What is a slow beauty mindset?

Slow beauty is a holistic approach to beauty and skincare. That means that slow beauty is part of an evaluation of choices that go beyond our skin and to the heart of how and why we buy.

If you are interested in slow beauty and minimalist skincare, then it is likely you are also thinking similarly about what you are eating and what clothes you buy.

Slow beauty is a mindset and a move towards a lifestyle of slower living.

Over consumption and a demand for newness has meant that the beauty industry has fallen into a continuous loop of new product development and "fast" beauty launches, which are synonymous with fast fashion.

Buying lots of new beauty products, purchasing the latest skincare trends and buying into the hype of beauty product launches has fuelled the rise of the shelfie, photos showing rows and rows of beauty, make-up or skincare products on people's bathroom shelves.

For a slow beauty consumer less is more.

Slowing down our beauty and skincare is about prioritising health and wellbeing. It is a change in perspective that encourages a more responsible and healthier standpoint.

What is a skinimalist?

Skinimalism, is a mash up term of skincare and minimalism. It is the ultimate no buy beauty, using less, buying slower and having minimal products in our bathroom cabinet.

Skinimalists are minimalist skincare users that believe using fewer products and fewer ingredients is better for our skin. Skinimalists use fewer products.

Skinimalists use fewer products on their skin. They may only use one, two or three products in total or they may use a small, curated range of products. They do not use multiple products a day nor do they have different products for morning, afternoon or evening.

Skinimalists stand in opposition to the endless hype of the beauty industry.

The beauty industry has become like fast fashion, there are fast beauty launches and trend led products developed to satisfy the constant need for newness. In a world of over consumption and weaker skin, consumers now seek a new kind of beauty, and that is minimalism.

What are the benefits of skinimalism?

Overuse of skincare products and ingredients are often responsible for damaging the skin barrier, which leads to an even greater reliance on multiple products. When we strip our skincare back to natural minimal ingredients from plants, the skin thrives.

More people than ever are experiencing thin skin, sensitive skin and weak skin.

Instead of using lots of products that can damage our skin, it is possible to have strong healthy skin with fewer skincare products.

Instead of ten step routines, skinimalists believe two steps can be enough. Instead of twenty skincare products in our drawer, skinimalists believe that three products can be enough.

Using fewer products is one thing but true skinimalists look to use fewer ingredients on their skin.

Lots of beauty brands deliberately take on a minimalist aesthetic, which can be misleading because when we read their ingredient lists their products are stuffed with ingredients. Skinimalists seek out products that have fewer highly effective ingredients (that work together to help the skin barrier be healthier).

6 Botanical Ingredients

Have you ever counted the number of ingredients listed on your skincare products? I did and found 20, 30, 40, even up to 100 in some cases.

I have a minimalist approach to skin care and believe fewer ingredients in your skin care is better for your overall skin barrier health.

This section takes a deep dive into some of the botanical ingredients we used when formulating our products at Five Dot Botanics and why we used them.

We only ever use five ingredients in any product we make

We make sure that what we use is effective and good for your skin.

I have included the common names of the botanical plants we work with; however you will also find the scientific name shown, which is the name you will see listed on the INCI list when you read our cosmetics label.

Amla oil / Indian Gooseberry oil

Scientific name: Phyllanthus Emblica (Amla) Fruit Extract
Comes from: the fruit and seeds

In Ayurvedic and traditional folk medicine throughout south-east Asia, this is one of the most important plants. It's had many scientific studies that have shown it to have antibacterial, antioxidant, and anti-inflammatory properties, making it multi-functional in a skincare product.

We use Amla oil in our Deep Feed facial serum.

Cacay nut oil

Scientific name: Caryodendron orinocense (Cacay) nut oil
Comes from: Nuts from the Cacay tree

Cacay oil is nutrient-dense, with a high content of natural Vitamin A, E, and F. It has 50% more Vitamin E and twice the amount of Linoleic Acid of Argan Oil. It also has a natural retinol, at three times the level of Rosehip Seed Oil. All these elements help it to restore skin's glow and vitality. When skin is well nourished, it looks smoother, and smoother skin always looks more vibrant.

We use Cacay in our Deep Feed facial serum.

Caffeine

Scientific name: Caffeine
Comes from: tea leaves and coffee beans

Caffeine has potent antioxidant properties, which help the skin to ward off the effects of pollution amongst other things. Pollution contributes to the level of free radicals on your skin. Antioxidants are one of the best ways of helping the skin fight them off. It also plays a role in slowing down the photo-ageing of your skin (the type that comes from being out and about).

We use caffeine in our Full Bright eye serum.

Carrot oil

Scientific name: Daucus Carota Sativa (Carrot) Root Extract
Comes from: Carrots (the orange bit as opposed to the tops)

Carrot oil is a vitamin-packed marvel. Carrot oil is extremely rich in beta-carotene, vitamins A, B, C, D, and E as well as essential fatty acids. The high beta-carotene content makes it particularly useful for dry skin.

We use Carrot oil in our Daily Prep facial oil.

Coffee seed oil

Scientific name: Coffea arabica (Coffee) seed oil
Comes from: green coffee beans

Coffee seed oil is known for its elevated levels of chlorogenic acid, another immensely powerful antioxidant, not to mention high levels of phytosterols. It has three times the levels of phytosterols as you'd find in green tea. When you combine those things with its combination of fatty acids, you've got something that helps the skin to retain moisture. It's been used for skin smoothing products, as well as for its skin calming properties.

We use coffee seed oil in our Deep Feed facial serum.

Evening primrose oil

Scientific name: Oenothera Biennis (Evening Primrose) Oil
Comes from Evening primrose seeds.

Evening Primrose is one of those almost legendary oils, beloved for everything from PMS to eczema. It contains Gamma linoleic acid, an essential fatty acid, and a crucial ingredient to healthy-looking skin. It's not just good for those of us with dry skin, but also if you've got oily skin, as your skin could still be short of linoleic acid. That can lead to thicker sebum, which blocks pores and leads to breakouts.

We use Evening Primrose in our Daily Prep facial oil.

Glycerin

Scientific name: Glycerin
Comes from: Usually from soya bean (but always vegetable derived in our products)

Used in different forms for many years, glycerin helps the skin to attract water, and then to hold onto it. You might see it listed as glycerine or glycerol, simply different spellings for the same thing. There are animal-derived versions, but we only ever use vegetable-derived versions.

We use glycerin in our Pure Rewind face mask, Calm Shift cleansing face balm, Full Bright eye serum and Brighten Up face mist.

Glycolipids

Scientific name: Glycolipids
Comes from: Sugar

Glycolipids are exceptionally mild and gentle when it comes to getting skin clean. This makes it suitable for every kind of skin. It's also 100% based on natural renewable ingredients (sugar), 100% biodegradable and contributes to the reduction of waste in natural water and marine ecosystems. It's exactly the kind of ingredient we want to be using: good for your skin, low impact on the planet.

We use glycolipids in our Pure Rewind face mask and Calm Shift cleansing balm.

Grapeseed oil

Scientific name: Vitis vinifera (Grape) seed oil
Comes from: Grape seeds

Grapeseed oil is a useful source of antioxidants to help your skin battle free radicals, which lead to premature signs of ageing. We're happy to age, but no one wants to do it prematurely! Helping the skin to control moisture, it's also been shown to have antibacterial and anti-inflammatory properties.

We grapeseed oil in our Daily Prep facial oil.

Hazelnut oil

Scientific name: Corylus Americana (Hazelnut) seed oil
Comes from: Hazelnuts

Hazelnut oil is packed with good things including oleic acid, linoleic acid, palmitic acid, and stearic acid. They all add up to an oil that's wonderfully conditioning for your skin.

We use hazelnut oil in our Calm Shift cleansing face balm

Horse Chestnut extract

Scientific name: Esculin
Comes from: seed, leaves and bark

We use horse chestnut for its action on soothing the skin and because it can help the microcirculation in your skin, which helps with things like reducing dark circle and undereye bags. It's also been shown to have wound healing properties. You will never look at a conker in the same way again.

We use horse chestnut in our Full Bright eye serum.

Lavender essential oil

Scientific name: Lavandula angustifolia (Lavender) oil
Comes from: leaves and flowering tops

Lavender essential oil is a bit of a legend. There's records of the ancient Persian, Romans and Greeks adding the flowers to their bathwater to help wash, purify, soften, and soothe skin. Lavender oil has been around for centuries, with people swearing by its calming and relaxing properties. But not only does it smell amazing, but it's also believed to have a whole host of skin benefits from anti-inflammatory to antibacterial.

We use lavender in our Pure Rewind face mask and Calm Shift cleansing face balm.

Levulinic Acid / Sodium Levulinate

Scientific name: Levulinic Acid; Sodium Levulinate

Where our formulas need to contain water, then there has to be a way of preserving them. This combination, found in many natural materials, has strong antibacterial properties, turning the formula into a self-preserving product. In fact, bees use this natural compound to protect the pollen and nectar from microbiological spoilage.

We use a Levulinic Acid and Sodium Levulinate mix in our Brighten Up face mist.

Liquorice root

Scientific name: Glycyrrhiza Glabra Root Extract
Comes from: the plant roots

We love liquorice, because the roots contain glycyrrhizic acid which has proved to have anti-inflammatory properties, as well as helping the skin's regeneration processes. It's a bit of a multi-tasker, helping to soothe sensitised skin as well as helping skin to look smoother. The smoother the skin, the more youthful and awake you look.

We use liquorice root in our Full Bright eye serum

Pomegranate enzymes

Scientific name: Lactobacillus/Punica Granatum Fruit Ferment Extract
Comes from: fruit pulp and fermenting the fruit extract with Lactobacillus lactis (a probiotic bacteria).

Pomegranate enzymes are a great alternative to alpha-hydroxy acids (AHA's), the pomegranate enzyme acts as a micro exfoliator. Gently removing the outer layer of dead skin cells, it helps your skin to look brighter and smoother. Those dead skin cells can also trap sebum and bacteria, making ideal conditions for breakouts. Regular, gentle exfoliation helps to keep everything clearer and brighter.

We use pomegranate enzymes in our Brighten Up face mist.

Rose clay

Scientific name: Kaolin (pink clay)
Comes from: the Mediterranean coast

This clay as a beautiful rosy-hue and helps to reduce irritation thanks to the sodium and potassium content. It's especially recommended for use in anti-stress treatments, which made it an ideal choice for our first face mask. It's got an unusually high absorption capacity, making it ideal for oily and combination skin.

We use rose clay in our Pure Rewind face mask.

Rose flower water

Scientific name: Rosa Damascena (Rose) flower water
Comes from: Damascus rose petals

Rose flower water is very gentle on your skin, it's been claimed that rosewater purifies and detoxifies as well as removing dirt and oil. It's also said to help stimulate blood circulation beneath the skin, which encourages new skin cell growth, and it helps to balance your skin's pH levels. It also has that beautiful delicate fragrance, which is a real mood-lifter for us.

We use rose water in our Brighten Up face mist.

Safflower seed oil

Scientific name: Carthamus Tinctorius (Safflower) Seed Oil
Comes from: Safflower seeds

Safflower seed oil is lightweight but packed with Linoleic and Oleic Acid, it's suitable for all skin types. It's believed to be anti-inflammatory, which can help your skin to feel calmer. Linoleic acid is thought to be able to mix with sebum which helps to unclog your pores and reduce blackheads. It makes it popular with people prone to acne and breakouts. It also helps to stimulate skin cell turnover, which in turn helps to clear up blemishes.

We use Safflower seed oil in both our Deep Feed facial serum and our Pure Rewind clay mask.

Sunflower oil

Scientific name: Helianthus annus (Sunflower) seed oil
Comes from: Sunflower seeds:

Sunflower oil helps your skin to stay hydrated for longer, thanks to its high vitamin E content. Studies have shown that Vitamin E in skincare products helps to protect the collagen and elastin in the skin. Think of them like your skin's bed springs. The better condition they're in, the bouncier and smoother your skin looks.

We use sunflower oil in our Daily Prep facial oil.

Sunflower seed wax

Scientific name: Helianthus Annus (Sunflower) Seed Wax
Comes from: Sunflower seeds

We use sunflower seed wax to give structure to our cleansing balm to help it melt onto your skin, this is one of the alternatives to using beeswax. As a vegan brand, we never use beeswax, and this gives us the melting properties we need to make the balm easy to melt and spread over your skin.
We use sunflower seed wax in our Calm Shift cleansing balm.

Ubuntu seed oil

Scientific name: Ximenia Americana (Ubuntu) Seed Oil
Comes from: Ubuntu seeds

Ubuntu seed oils is nourishing and moisturising, this oil naturally softens and revitalises your skin. When skin is well moisturised and hydrated, then it just looks more alive, more vibrant. Ubuntu seed oil is also a great natural alternative to silicones, giving that silky feel as you massage the product into your skin.

We Ubuntu seed in our Daily Prep facial oil.

ABOUT THE AUTHOR

Zaffrin O'Sullivan is co-founder of British minimal ingredient skincare brand Five Dot Botanics.

She is a lawyer turned beauty entrepreneur. She is also the founder of beauty community, Female Founders in Beauty.

She lives in London with her husband and three children.

ABOUT FIVE DOT BOTANICS

Five Dot Botanics makes award-winning minimal ingredient skincare that helps to protect, repair, and nourish the skin barrier.

Everything in the range is designed for skin health, using only five natural ingredients from plants.

Five Dot Botanics offers effective gentle skincare without a complicated ingredients list. Their ethos is that fewer ingredients in skincare is better for your skin barrier health and better for the planet.

Vegan certified. Cruelty free. Made in Britain.

www.fivedotbotanics.com

@fivedotbotanics

Index

A
Amla oil / Indian Gooseberry oil **133**

Are AHAs and enzymes the only chemical exfoliants? **104**

Are common allergens listed on the INCI? **75**

Are cosmetics tested on animals? **83**

Are enzymes better than acids? **105**

Are skincare products biodegradable? **85**

B
Botanical Ingredients **132**

C
Cacay nut oil **133**

Caffeine **133**

Carrot oil **134**

Coffee seed oil **134**

D
Decode Your Skincare **93**

Deepest layer **5**

Do cosmetic products get absorbed beyond the skin? **97**

Does skin differ between gender? **40**

Does the order of applying skincare products

matter? **53**

Does the skin renew itself? **27**

Do men and women need to use different skincare products? **40**

E
Evening primrose oil **135**

G
Glycerin **135**

Glycolipids **136**

Grapeseed oil **136**

H
Hazelnut oil **136**

Horse Chestnut extract **137**

How can exercise help skin health? **122**

How can I tell if my skincare product is vegan? **79**

How can we protect the acid mantle? **19**

How can you avoid parabens? **109**

How do adaptogens benefit skin? **107**

How do companies test their skincare products? **89**

How does cleansing help other products? **48**

How does our gut health impact our skin? **121**

How does skin age? **24**

How does sleep improve our skin? **117**

How does stress effect our skin? **115**

How does the microbiome help our skin? **22**

How does the sun affect skin? **37**

How does the sun cause oxidative stress? **38**

How does trans-epidermal water loss (TEWL) effect skin? **62**

How do I build a skincare routine? **44**

How do I cleanse? **46**

How do I know if my acid mantle is damaged? **18**

How do I protect my skin barrier? **11**

How is skin care self-care? **122**

How is the skin barrier damaged? **7**

How many cosmetic products do you use a day? **71**

How to keep skin healthy while wearing a face mask? **66**

How to practice slow beauty? **127**

How to think of your skin care holistically? **114**

How to treat dehydrated skin? **63**

How to use a gua sha tool for face massage? **125**

I
Is the acid mantle related to skin's pH? **15**

L
Lavender essential oil **137**

Levulinic Acid / Sodium Levulinate **138**

Liquorice root **138**

M
Middle layer **5**

O
Other Skin Conditions **35**

Outer layer **4**

P
Pomegranate enzymes **138**

R
Rose clay **139**

Rose flower water **139**

S
Safflower seed oil **140**

Should you avoid fragrance in your skincare? **109**

Should you avoid parabens? **108**

Skin Basics **1**

Skin Care **42**

Skin & Wellness **112**

Sunflower oil **140**

Sunflower seed wax **141**

T
The difference between natural skin care and organic skin care? **83**

U
Ubuntu seed oil **141**

W
What animal ingredients are in skincare? **106**

What are AHAs? **103**

What are enzymes? **104**

What are microbiome skin care products? **23**

What are microplastics? **86**

What are non-comedogenic products? **88**

What are parabens used for? **108**

What are skin conditions? **31**

What are skin types? **29**

What are the benefits of a good diet on our skin? **119**

What are the benefits of exfoliation? **49**

What are the benefits of having a skin care routine? **42**

What are the benefits of skinimalism? **130**

What are the benefits of using a clay mask? **60**

What are the main layers of the skin? **4**

What are the signs of skin barrier damage? **10**

What are the skin benefits of drinking water? **118**

What can we do to help manage stress? **117**

What causes dark eye circles? **36**

What does 'clean' skincare mean? **76**

What does our skin do? **3**

What factors affect skin pH? **17**

What happens if cosmetics are not preserved? **89**

What happens when our microbiome is out of balance? **23**

What is a basic evening routine? **55**

What is a basic morning routine? **54**

What is a cosmetic? **70**

What is a facial oil? **58**

What is an INCI list? **74**

What is a safety assessment? **91**

What is a skinimalist? **129**

What is a slow beauty mindset? **128**

What is CBD skincare? **110**

What is cleansing? **45**

What is combination skin? **30**

What is cruelty free beauty? **84**

What is difference between chemical and physical exfoliants? **51**

What is dry skin? **30**

What is face yoga? **127**

What is green chemistry in skincare? **87**

What is green washing? **87**

What is happening to skin in our fifties onward? **27**

What is happening to skin in our forties? **26**

What is happening to skin in our thirties? **26**

What is happening to skin in our twenties? **26**

What is holistic skin care? **113**

What is maskne? **65**

What is meant by synthetic ingredients in skincare? **95**

What is microbiological testing? **91**

What is minimalist skincare? **80**

What is my skin type? **30**

What is natural skin care? **94**

What is normal skin? **30**

What is oily skin? **31**

What is organic skincare? **83**

What is oxidative stress? **102**

What is retinol? **61**

What is Skin? **4**

What is stability testing? **90**

What is sustainable skincare? **84**

What is the benefit of using a gua sha tool? **125**

What is the difference between hemp and CBD? **111**

What is the difference between mineral oils and plant oils? **99**

What is the difference between moisturising and hydrating? **53**

What is the difference between vegan and cruelty-free products? **79**

What is the meaning of certified organic? **83**

What is the skin barrier? **6**

What is the skin microbiome? **21**

What is the skin's acid mantle? **14**

What is vegan skincare? **78**

What is waterless beauty? **81**

What things are listed on a skincare label? **72**

When did the beauty industry start? **69**

When to use a face mask? **59**

Who are AHAs best suited to? **104**

Who are enzymes best suited to? **105**

Why are facial workouts good? **123**

Why choose natural skincare? **95**

Why does skin feel different in winter? **64**

Why do we get wrinkles? **39**

Why do we need to hydrate? **51**

Why is palm oil used in skincare? **100**

Why is skin important? **2**

Why is skin microbiome important? **21**

Why is skin pH important to skin health? **16**

Why read skincare labels? **72**

Why try facial massage? **126**

Why we need a hydrating mist? **48**

Why you need an SPF? **62**

Why you should avoid sheet masks? **60**

Printed in Great Britain
by Amazon